Mouth Actions in Sign Languages

Sign Languages and Deaf Communities 3

De Gruyter Mouton · Ishara Press

Mouth Actions in Sign Languages

An Empirical Study of Irish Sign Language

By
Susanne Mohr

De Gruyter Mouton · Ishara Press

ISBN 978-1-61451-705-4
e-ISBN 978-1-61451-497-8
ISSN 2192-516X
e-ISSN 2192-5178

Library of Congress Cataloging-in-Publication Data

A CIP catalog record for this book has been applied for at the Library of Congress.

Bibliographic information published by the Deutsche Nationalbibliothek

The Deutsche Nationalbibliothek lists this publication in the Deutsche Nationalbibliografie; detailed bibliographic data are available in the Internet at http://dnb.dnb.de.

Printing and binding: CPI books GmbH, Leck
♾ Printed on acid-free paper

Printed in Germany

www.degruyter.com

Acknowledgements

Many people have accompanied this book in its development from a raw manuscript to the edited book. I couldn't have finished it without them and I want to express my gratitude to them here.

First of all, my deepest thanks go to my PhD supervisor, Silvia Kutscher. Thank you for taking me on as a PhD student, for supporting me academically and personally in situations when this whole endeavour seemed at stake. I appreciate your comments on my texts, they helped me see several linguistic problems clearer.

I would also like to thank all the people who were involved in the editing, production and printing process of this book. Markus Steinbach, Ulrike Zeshan and Annika Herrmann for editorial insights and support. Thank you for always being available for even the tiniest questions relating to the text and the publishing process. Thanks also to Nicola Wright for production and final compilation of the book, as well as to Emily Farrell at de Gruyter Mouton.

For scholarly criticism and linguistic advice, thanks to my anonymous reviewer. This book was very much improved by your expertise in sign languages and linguistics and the attentive eye you turned on the manuscript.

Thank you to the a.r.t.e.s. Graduate School for the Humanities Cologne for financial as well as academic support. It is a privilege to receive a PhD scholarship in Germany. I especially appreciate the feedback I got from Claudia Riehl. Thank you for supporting me and my work – and for the discussions in class and on your balcony.

A big thank you goes to Lorraine Leeson and the Centre for Deaf Studies at Trinity College, Dublin. Thank you for giving me the opportunity to work with the ISL data, for supporting me during my trip to Dublin in 2009 and beyond. For answering all my small and bigger questions. Without your expertise on ISL, this wouldn't have been possible.

Further, thank you to all the signers who agreed that their data be published. Caroline W., Eilish B., Fergus D., Fergus M., Kevin L., Laurence H., Marian H., Michelle M., Noeleen D., Peter M., Sarah-Jane M. and Sean H.

Thank you to my proof-readers: Aaron Horton and Vanessa Crouch for native speaker support, I could always rely on your expertise of the English language. I am also indebted to Anastasia Bauer, Anne Fehn, Kirsten Gather and Maxi Limbach who (re-)read rather long parts of this book and helped me improve it with their comments.

There is only one group of people left that I haven't mentioned yet: my family and friends. You all supported me morally, especially in believing in me and my work no matter what. Thank you for countless talks over the phone, over hot tea or a pint, for emails and letters.

Contents

Acknowledgements v

List of figures xi

List of tables xiv

Abbreviations xv

Notational Conventions xvii

1. Introduction 1

2. The Linguistic Setup of Sign Languages – The Case of Irish Sign Language (ISL) 4

   2.1. The Sociolinguistics of ISL 5

   2.2. The Educational System and Oralism 9

   2.3. Structural Issues: The Use of Space 11

   2.4. Structural Issues: Iconicity 18

   2.5. Structural Issues: Simultaneity 21

   2.6. Structural issues: Non-manual Features 24

3. Non-manuals in Sign Languages – Theoretical Background 31

   3.1. Non-Mouth Related Non-Manuals 32

      3.1.1. Eye Gaze 32

      3.1.2. Facial Expression 34

         3.1.2.1. Facial Expression and the Lexicon 35

         3.1.2.2. Facial Expression and Syntax 36

         3.1.2.3. Facial Expression and Prosody 46

      3.1.3. Head Movements 48

3.2. Mouth Actions 50
3.2.1. Mouth Gestures 51
3.2.2. Echo Phonology 54
3.2.3. Mouthings 55
3.2.4. Spreading of Mouth Actions 61

4. Mouth Actions in ISL – A Typology of Mouthings and Mouth Gestures 64
4.1. Data Sources and Methodology 66
4.2. Categorization of Mouth Actions in the SOI Data 71
4.2.1. Mouthings 71
4.2.2. Mouth Gestures 84
4.2.3. Mouth Actions in the SOI at a Glance 92

5. Mouth Actions in ISL – Sociolinguistic Factors 94
5.1. Research Questions and Hypotheses 94
5.2. Mouth Actions and Gender 95
5.2.1. Mouth Actions in Women 95
5.2.2. Mouth Actions in Men 97
5.2.3. Comparison of Mouth Actions in Men and Women 99
5.3. Combining Two Sociolinguistic Factors – Gender and Age 102

6. Mouth Actions in ISL – Linguistic Factors 114
6.1. Word Classes – Historical and Theoretical Background 115
6.1.1. Semantic Approaches to Word Class Distinction 118
6.1.2. Syntactic Approaches to Word Class Distinction 122
6.1.3. Morphosyntactic Approaches to Word Class Distinction 123
6.1.4. Word Class Distinction in Sign Languages 126
6.1.5. Discussion 131

6.2. Mouth Actions and Word Classes in ISL 132
6.2.1. Syntactic Categories of ISL 134
6.2.2. Lexical Classes of ISL 138
6.2.3. Correlations of Word Classes and Mouth Actions 144
6.2.4. Mouth Gestures as a Category in Its Own Right? 148
6.2.5. Discussion of the Results within a Functional Linguistic Model 154
7. Conclusion 162

Appendix A
Complete list of lexical signs and fingerspellings with mouthings........... 166

Appendix B
Contexts for examples (glossed with mouthings).................................... 185

Notes 204

Reference 212

Index 228

List of figures

2.1	St. Mary's School for Deaf Girls, Cabra	10
2.2	St. Joseph's School for Deaf Boys, Cabra	10
2.3	The signing space	12
2.4	Locations of singular person agreement in the signing space	14
2.5	The ISL sign ASK inflecting for person	15
2.6	Person inflection in ISL signs	16
2.7	The ISL sign MOCK	17
2.8	The ISL sign FLY	17
2.9	The ISL sign KEY	20
2.10	ISL PRO_1-GIVE-CYLINDRICAL-OBJECT (glass)-PRO_2	20
2.11	The ISL sign MINICOM	24
2.12	The ISL signs COLD and COLDER	25
2.13	The ISL signs WARY/DISBELIEF/UNSURE and FALSE	25
2.14	The ISL signs for 'Who?', 'Who!' and 'you are not who I think you are!'	26
2.15	'It was difficult to get through the crowd.'	27
2.16	The ISL signs WHO, WHEN and WHERE	28
2.17	ISL for 'I don't understand' including a negation particle	29
2.18	ISL for 'I don't understand' without a negation particle	29
2.19	CAMERA INDEX MINE – 'That camera is mine'	30
3.1	Hierarchy of non-manuals	31
3.2	BSL signs GOD and BOSS	33
3.3	LSC signs PITY and FALL-IN-LOVE	36
3.4	Grammatical facial expression in ASL: Statement	37
3.5	Grammatical facial expression in ASL: Question	37
3.6	Grammatical facial expression in ASL: Relative clause	38

3.7	tm1 for ASL	41
3.8	tm2 for ASL	41
3.9	tm3 and alternative version for ASL	41
3.10	The use of facial expression in conditional clauses in DGS	44
3.11	IsSL signs I and I-READ	48
4.1	Manner markers in ISL	65
4.2	Map of Ireland	67
4.3	Typical ELAN file from the SOI	68
4.4	TYPE 1 mouthing	72
4.5	TYPE 2 mouthing	72
4.6	TYPE 3a mouthing	73
4.7	TYPE 3b mouthing	73
4.8	TYPE 4 mouthing	75
4.9	TYPE 5 mouthing	76
4.10	TYPE 6a mouthing	77
4.11	TYPE 6b mouthing	79
4.12	TYPE 6c mouthing	81
4.13	Fingerspelling and mouthing combination	84
4.14	Adverbial mouth gesture 1	85
4.15	Adverbial mouth gesture 2	86
4.16	Adverbial mouth gesture 3	87
4.17	Adverbial mouth gesture 4	87
4.18	Semantically empty mouth gesture 1	87
4.19	Semantically empty mouth gesture 2	88
4.20	Semantically empty mouth gesture 3	89
4.21	Enacting mouth gesture 1	90
4.22	Enacting mouth gesture 2	90
4.23	Enacting mouth gesture 3	91

5.1 Mismatch of the manual sign BICYCLE and the mouthing "ladder" 97
5.2 Comparison of mouth actions in men and women 100
5.3 Spreading directions in men and women 101
5.4 Comparison of mouth actions across age groups 102
5.5 Comparison of mouth actions in men and women in age group 1 105
5.6 Comparison of mouth actions in men and women in age group 2 105
5.7 Comparison of mouth actions in men and women in age group 3 106
5.8 Comparison of mouth actions for all sociolinguistic factors 108

6.1 Inflectional ending in Signed English 136
6.2 Relation of lexical classes and syntactic categories in ISL 144
6.3 Correlation between mouth actions and syntactic categories in ISL 145
6.4 Correlation between mouth actions and lexical classes in ISL 147
6.5 Correlation between mouth actions and verbal subclasses in ISL 148
6.6 The ISL sign PLAY-HARD-AGAINST-EACH-OTHER 151
6.7 The ISL sign THROW-DOWN-SHOVEL 152
6.8 The ISL sign WHISPER-IN-EAR 153
6.9 Dik's model of functional grammar 159

List of tables

4.1 Signers chosen for the analysis of mouth actions in ISL 69

5.1 Mouthings in women 96

5.2 Mouthings in men 98

5.3 Correlation of mouthings and language of family communication during childhood 111

Abbreviations

AdaSL	Adamorobe Sign Language
ASL	American Sign Language
Auslan	Australian Sign Language
BENEF	Benefective marker
BSL	British Sign Language
CL	Classifier
CSL	Chinese Sign Language
DGS	Deutsche Gebärdensprache = German Sign Language
DISTR	Distributive aktionsart
DSGS	Deutschschweizer Gebärdensprache = Swiss-German Sign Language
DSL	Danish Sign Language
HKSL	Hong Kong Sign Language
hs	headshake
HSL	Hausa Sign Language
INT	Intensive aktionsart
Int	Intonationational Phrase
IPSL	Indopakistani Sign Language
ISL	Irish Sign Language
IsSL	Israeli Sign Language
IT	Iterative aktionsart
LBG	Lautsprachbegleitende Gebärden = Signed German
LIS	Lingua dei Segni Italiana = Italian Sign Language

LOC	Locative marker
LSC	Llengua des Signes Catalana = Catalan Sign Language
LSF	Langue des Signes Française = French Sign Language
LSQ	Langue des Signes Québécois = Quebec Sign Language
MSL	Mauritian Sign Language
NGT	Nederlandse Gebaarental = Dutch Sign Language
NSL	Norwegian Sign Language
PERF	Perfective marker
PL	Plural marker
PoS	Part(s)-of-speech
POSS	Possessive marker
PRO	Pronoun
re	raised eyebrows
RPRO	Relative pronoun
SASL	South African Sign Language
SG	Singular
SOI	Signs of Ireland Corpus
SSL	Swedish Sign Language
tm	Topic marker
TSL	Turkish Sign Language
wh	Non-manual for wh-questions

Notational Conventions

As many linguists are not acquainted with the notational conventions for sign languages, they are explained briefly here. Even within the domain of sign linguistics, there is no universally valid convention for sign language transcription. The notational system used in this book is mainly oriented on Prillwitz's (1985) and Klima/Bellugi's (1979) notation of sign sequences.

he-**OWN**	Sign language glosses are written in capitals. These capitalized glosses refer to the picture of a sign (sequence) as it would be shown in an ELAN screenshot. While sometimes these pictures are actually provided, due to space restrictions this was not possible for all glosses. Lower case letters before or after a gloss indicate additional meanings which are contained in the manual sign. They are joined by a hyphen.
question ? you-**OWN**	The upper line of a sentence transcription conveys information on non-manuals like facial expression, movement of the body or mouth actions. They are uttered simultaneously with the manual sign. e.g. question (interrogative) negation affirmation duration etc. The line before the non-manual marker indicates which signs are accompanied by the respective marker. Mouthings are notated in English orthography while mouth gestures are notated using the ECHO conventions which are descriptive of the mouth movements. Although I am aware that mouthings are sometimes notated as phonetic transcripts, I decided against this option, as mouthings are usually voiceless so a system representing the sounds of a language seemed inappropriate here.

INDEX-	This symbol marks a manual sign formed by the index finger. References, i.e. referential loci are thus established within the sign space. Additional information like P_1 added before or after the hyphen, refers to the system of referential person loci in the signing space.
THREE-WEEK	Hyphenated glosses indicate that only one manual sign is formed to express both meanings expressed in the gloss. The meanings of both glosses are merged in one single manual sign.
DRIVE+	A + behind a gloss stands for repetition or reduplication of the whole sign or its movement path. The number of + indicates the number of repetitions of the gloss.
(DA)	Glosses in parentheses could be left out.
d.r.i.v.e.	Fingerspelt words are represented by letters separated by dots.
DRIVE//RIDE	Glosses separated by slashes are part of a compound and are signed in quick succession.
'drive'	Words in single quotes indicate a) a non-conventionalised sign if they are on the same level as the sign language gloss, or b) the semantic meaning of a sign or sentence if below gloss level.

It should be mentioned that other researchers sometimes annotated their data differently. Diverging notations that are found throughout the text (especially with reference to mouth actions) are:

<u>**MOUNTAIN**</u>	Underlined glosses represent manual signs that are accompanied by the mouthed spoken word.
BESITZEN *sch*	Single letters beneath a gloss indicate mouthed sounds different from the mouthed gloss.

Chapter 1
Introduction

Sign languages are languages of the hands. While this is probably what most people and even linguists associate with sign languages, it is not consistent with linguistic reality. Although it is certainly true that sign languages are visual-gestural languages in which the hands and manual signs play an important role in conveying meaning, there are other articulators that are equally important. Kutscher (2007) mentions three types of signs:

1. Manual signs
2. Signs of the mouth, head and torso
3. Voiceless words of the surrounding spoken language, formed with the mouth

As becomes clear from the list above, there are other major articulators apart from the hands. The signs formed by these articulators are usually called "non-manuals" and include actions of the mouth. While non-manuals in general and mouth actions in particular were rather neglected in the beginning of sign linguistic research, the past two decades have brought forth an increasing number of in-depth studies of non-manuals in various sign languages. Mouth actions and the generally assumed dichotomy of "signs of the mouth" and "voiceless words of the surrounding spoken language" that are mentioned above remain an under-researched and controversial topic. For Irish Sign Language (ISL), used in the Republic and Northern Ireland, this topic has not been researched empirically as yet. This book constitutes the first systematic analysis of the structure and dynamics of these kinds of non-manuals. The main topics discussed in this study will be elaborated in the next section.

The main research question underlying this analysis is whether the general dichotomy of mouth actions that has been established for other sign languages can be found in ISL and whether these mouth actions are used systematically. Further, it will be investigated whether mouth actions fulfill specific linguistic functions and if so, what the nature of these functions is. It will be especially interesting to look at the voiceless words of the surrounding spoken language (also called "mouthings" in the literature (Boyes Braem & Sutton-Spence 2001)), as these have been a highly controversial topic in sign linguistics thus far. While they are frequently found and used in some sign languages with a strong oral tradition in education such as German Sign Language (DGS), for example, they are said to be absent from or rarely used in others such as American Sign Language (ASL). Moreover, it has frequently been claimed that they do not form part of the linguistic system of a sign language and could be discarded (e.g. Happ & Hohenberger 2001). This claim will be tested with respect to ISL.

Concerning the other type of mouth actions (also called "mouth gestures" in the literature (Boyes Braem & Sutton-Spence 2001)), it will be interesting to see whether the same subtypes that have been found for other sign languages such as Dutch Sign Language (NGT), can be found in ISL.

With special reference to the linguistic and sociolinguistic situation of ISL, there are additional research questions that are relevant. One of the most prominent features of ISL is the striking gender difference at the linguistic and paralinguistic level. This can be traced back to gender segregation in schooling (cf. chapters 2.1 and 2.2). It will therefore be interesting to investigate whether these gender differences can also be observed with respect to mouth actions. Age is another sociolinguistic factor that has been mentioned as being relevant for linguistic variation in ISL (Ó Baoill & Matthews 2000). Consequently, the influence of this factor on mouth actions will be analyzed as well. Referring to linguistic factors, word class or morphological complexity have been mentioned to be interrelated with the use of mouth actions (e.g. Crasborn et al. 2008). Therefore, this claim will be examined in conjunction with the ISL data, too.

In order to answer the aforementioned research questions, the book is structured as follows. Chapter 2 provides a short outline of Irish Sign Language and its sociolinguistics, as well as general structural characteristics. This will be useful for interested linguists who do not possess further knowledge of sign languages and their structures. Chapter 3 introduces non-manuals in sign languages from a cross-linguistic point of view. Differences and similarities in form and function of these non-manuals are outlined; a special focus is on mouth actions as the main focus of this volume. In chapter 4, the data sources and methodology applied to the language data from ISL are introduced. In the second part of the chapter, a general typology of mouth actions with respect to the SOI data is introduced. Chapter 5 investigates the influence of sociolinguistic factors on mouth actions in ISL and describes the interrelations between mouth actions and gender and age in ISL. Chapter 6 constitutes the second empirical chapter of this book. In order to make the investigation of the interrelation between mouth actions and word classes more comprehensible, the first part of the chapter shortly sketches the history and theoretical framework of word class research in spoken and sign languages. The second part of the chapter provides the analysis of the data with respect to this issue and situates the analysis in a grammatical framework. Chapter 7 summarizes the results of the study and provides some concluding remarks.

Chapter 2
The Linguistic Setup of Sign Languages – The Case of Irish Sign Language (ISL)

ISL is a primary sign language and the native language of the approximately 6,500 deaf people living in the Republic and Northern Ireland, although British Sign Language (BSL) is used frequently in the latter. ISL is genetically closely related to French Sign Language (LSF), although BSL has had a major impact on the language due to televised BSL programmes, the migration of deaf people to the UK and co-operations of Deaf organizations in Ireland and the UK (Leeson & Grehan 2004). The exact origin of ISL is unknown, as the grammar of the language remains undocumented prior to the establishment of deaf schools in Ireland, starting around 1814 (Matthews 1996).

Although the above reads like a short sketch of any other (spoken) language in the world that is more or less well documented and whose language family and linguistic typology have been analyzed, it is rather exceptional in the fields of sign linguistics and sign language typology. Actually, only a minority of the world's (sign) languages has been documented so far and even fewer works have treated the typology of signed languages[1] (Wilkinson 2009). The fact that Zeshan in 2008 still discusses the novelty of the field of sign language typology as well as possible methods, emphasizes the paucity of studies and knowledge about sign language typology. However, this is not surprising given that only a few sign languages have been documented so far and, even for those sign languages that have been studied, an imbalance towards Western sign languages persists. Most studies in sign linguistics focus on ASL and Western European sign languages. Other types, such as non-Western urban sign languages and village sign languages, have been rarely studied and only came to the attention of the sign linguistic community in recent works like Nyst (2007; 2012), Schwager and Zeshan (2008). Studies like these have revealed the falsity of some claims about the universality of certain linguistic features of signed languages. The use of space and spatial time lines that were believed to exist in all sign languages and have been proven not to, is only one example. A broader knowledge of the genealogy of signed languages (of which only little is known) or the different types of sign languages in the world might help to solve typological questions related to sign languages, which remain very controversial to date.

Central issues of sign language typology refer to two different domains: general linguistics and sign linguistics. Neither a sub-classification nor a typology of the "sign language family", nor a typological classification of sign languages on morphological grounds as either isolating, fusional, agglutinating or polysynthetic has yet been achieved. Apparently, a curious mix of grammatical phenomena prevents a clear morphological categorization of signed languages into one of the established types of spoken languages. This clearly shows that more research on sign language grammar is necessary, even more so given that new insights into sign language typology will further linguists' knowledge of linguistic structures in general.

Having experienced that most spoken language linguists are not acquainted with sign language structures, subsequent sections will provide an overview of the grammar of sign languages, tackling some of the issues in sign language typology. All sections especially focus on ISL. The first part of the chapter provides an introduction to the language: it concentrates on the sociolinguistic situation and the status of ISL in Ireland. A description of deaf education and its history in Ireland will also be provided, as it is crucial for the analysis of the data from the Signs of Ireland Corpus. In the second part, grammatical features that have been found for all sign language systems studied so far will be discussed. This outline includes a sketch of non-manual features in ISL, of which mouth actions are a part.

2.1. The Sociolinguistics of ISL

ISL, although Ireland's second native language along with Irish, still has no official status in Irish legislation despite EU resolutions (e.g. 1998) and the Council of Europe Parliamentary Assembly (2003) (Leeson 2008). Just like other minority languages in Ireland, such as Gammon or Cant, spoken by the Irish Travellers, it has no legal status in the constitution, perhaps due to the fact that Ireland is not a traditionally multilingual country. Attempts at raising the official status of ISL as well as that of other sign languages are constantly being made but only very few of them are successful. To date, Sweden, South Africa and Brazil remain some of the few countries to have officially acknowledged their national sign languages as one of the official languages of the country (Reagan 2010).

As minority languages, sign languages around the world are subject to problems similar to spoken minority languages. Moreover, the fact that only 5% of all deaf children are born to deaf parents and thus acquire a sign language in a family environment instead of a school, adds to the array of obstacles these languages have to overcome. Traditional transmission, or rather the lack thereof, is often mentioned as one of the main criteria that lead to language endangerment (e.g. Brenzinger 2007; Drossard 2009). Furthermore, almost all of the nine UNESCO criteria that have a major impact on language endangerment apply to sign languages and their environment. Plaza Pust (2005) mentions that in the case of deaf communities, language planning and language policies are particularly critical because the minority language and the majority language do not represent equal codes for deaf individuals.

Generally, there is no standard way by which the legal recognition of a sign language is realized. Thus, it could be acknowledged as one of the official languages of a country in the country's constitution. Sometimes, sign languages have a special status in education, a fact that is apparent in the use of the national sign language in schools for the deaf. Hence, DGS or LBG[2] are used in most German deaf schools as the medium of instruction. Plaza Pust (2005) also mentions that deaf education in Europe is in a transitional stage characterized by a diversification of educational methods. This hints at the fact that to date, there is no consistency concerning the methods and especially the languages used in deaf education. While in many countries there are only a few schools with bilingual programmes for deaf children, such schools have been institutionalized in Scandinavia.

In Ireland, ISL is minimally present in the media through special ISL programmes such as "Hands On" on RTÉ One.[3] However, there are quite a number of deaf organizations such as the Irish Deaf Society or the Irish Deaf Youth Association. Moreover, ISL can be studied at the Centre for Deaf Studies at Trinity College Dublin where different courses at undergraduate and postgraduate levels are available. These include courses such as ISL/ English Interpreting, ISL teaching or Deaf Studies all of which are available to hearing and deaf students alike. Also, a project realizing the "neighbour method" proposed for endangered languages by Tsunoda (2006), e.g., is currently being carried out. The method suggests the establishment of settlements (villages, towns, cities) in which all members of a speech community live side by side and exclusively communicate in the endangered language. Hence, "Deaf Village Ireland" was opened in August 2012 in Cabra, Dublin. Several facilities as well as organizations can be found in the village, such as a sports centre, a chapel, offices for *Deaf Sports Ireland*, the Deaf Scouts, etc. To date, older Deaf people do not visit the village very often, as it is less conveniently located than Drumcondra, the part of Dublin that used to be the centre of Deaf activities (Gilchrist, pers. comm.). However, it is quite popular with younger Deaf people, so it remains to be seen whether older people will accept the village as a new Deaf centre as well.

As in most other deaf societies, deaf people in Ireland usually grow up bilingual (English/ISL). Often, ISL is not a signer's native language because s/he is born to hearing parents who do not know any ISL so that the child's first language is English. Only later in life (in school, for example) do they learn ISL. There are only very few deaf societies in the world in which the situation is the other way around. An example of this is Kata Kolok, the sign language of a village community in Bali, Indonesia, where a high incidence of hereditary deafness has led to the whole village knowing the sign language and being bilingual. In this case, deaf people in Kata Kolok are monolingual only, so the hearing people have to know the sign language alongside their spoken languages (Schwager & Zeshan 2008).[4]

Linguistic variation is a prominent feature of ISL, however, this can mostly be observed along gender lines due to traditional segregation in schooling, as will be discussed in section 2.2. The most important thing to remember for the moment is that distinct male-female varieties existed in ISL which were similar to distinct varieties found in some spoken languages such as Bambara (a Manding language of the Niger-Congo phylum), for instance.[5] Traces of these distinct varieties are still found in current signers' vocabularies (Ó Baoill & Matthews 2000; Leeson & Grehan 2004), especially in women's language use as the former male variety developed into standard ISL. Particularly, Le Master has investigated the differences between male and female ISL in numerous publications which focus mainly on the lexicon of ISL. Thus, according to Le Master (1990), there are related and unrelated sign groups in male and female signs. The related signs share certain formative features like handshapes or movement patterns, e.g., whereas the unrelated signs do not resemble each other in form. The terms "related" and "unrelated" signs usually refer to signs of different sign languages. Relation can thus be established on the basis of the formal properties of handshape, location and movement. Cognates are identical in all three features; related or similar signs overlap in two features and different signs are diverging in two or more features (Wilkinson 2009). These criteria are also applied when signs are compared on the basis of the modified Swadesh list for sign languages (Woodward 1978).[6] With respect to ISL, Le Master also mentions that the female variety was less initialized than the male one, i.e. that in the female variety there were less signs that were formed with a handshape taken from the manual alphabet of this sign language and representing the first letter of the corresponding English word.[7] Moreover, she mentions that the varieties were mutually unintelligible and that men and women had to learn the variety of the opposite sex. This issue is rather controversial, however, as other researchers mention, the different varieties never hampered communication among deaf people themselves.

Today, male and female varieties cannot be distinguished anymore. The male variety developed into present day ISL which is learnt by men and women alike. Many women, however, still use distinct lexical signs (cf. chapter 4). Recent publications, such as Leeson and Grehan (2004) mention gender differences on other linguistic levels such as the discourse level, for example. They investigated the form of topic-comment structures in ISL as well as the use of certain simultaneous constructions which turned out to be used differently by men and women (Leeson & Grehan 2004:68). Ó Baoill and Matthews (2000:14) mention that the style of female signing is dependent on the interlocutor's sex. Hence, women use a reduced signing space, the length or duration of signs is reduced and lexical choices differ from the ones made when communicating with a male signer. When signing in a mixed group, women tend to adjust their lexical choices to the male variety while men do not accommodate the female signs. Thus, gender differences have been found to exist in present day ISL and to permeate the lexical level.

There are also different registers of ISL, i.e. that a signer adjusts his language to different situations (Ó Baoill & Matthews 2000). The male variety is generally considered to be more formal and more standard by both sexes. This might be due to the fact that the former male variety developed into standard ISL, while it does in no way entail that male ISL signers use a more formal speech style in all situations of everyday life. Regional variation has not been reported yet and has also been claimed to be inexistent (Ó Baoill & Matthews 2000). However, more recent publications such as Leeson and Grehan (2004:39) mention that a) there might be a distinct Northern Irish variety of ISL which has however not been researched yet and b) regional variation might develop due to more and more deaf children being sent to partially deaf units at local schools instead of being sent to one of the deaf schools in Dublin. This has not been researched so far either.

In summary, ISL is a minority language that has not been acknowledged officially in the constitution, despite several attempts at promoting the language by national deaf organizations, for instance. Consequently, most deaf children in Ireland grow up bilingual and must have at least some knowledge of English. Sociolinguistic variation in ISL exists especially concerning gender, while situational variation is present, too, and regional variation between Northern Ireland and the Republic is assumed to be existent but has never been researched thus far.

2.2. The Educational System and Oralism

Formal deaf education in Ireland, as mentioned earlier, started at the beginning of the 19th century, with the establishment of the first schools (Matthews 1996[8]). In 1814, Dr. Charles Orpen, a medical doctor, became aware of the lack of any educational institution for the deaf when he returned from England, where this kind of institution had just been founded in Birmingham. Starting with only one student whom he took from an orphanage in Dublin, he began to research and publish on the matter of deaf education, leading ultimately to the establishment of a school in the Smithfield Penitentiary, Dublin, in 1816. In the beginning, six to eight boys attended; this number rose to 16, of which the majority were boarders. The school moved several times until its headmaster became head of the Claremont school (established in 1819) which, due to its large dimensions, became known as the "Irish National Institution for the Deaf and Dumb".

Several other schools were founded around the country, but many of them had to close after a few years due to falling numbers of students. A big problem in Catholic Ireland was the fact that Claremont was a Protestant co-educational school that taught its (mostly Catholic students) in the Protestant faith. Thus, in 1822, St. Mary's School in Cork was established by the physician Dr. Kehoe. This took place after Reverend Thomas McNamara had founded the Catholic Committee, a committee established due to his fear for the souls of the Catholic deaf children. As a co-educational school, St. Mary's had a total of 73 pupils until it closed down in 1846 due to lack of funding.

In 1845, Reverend Monsignor Yore established the first committee of the Catholic Institution for the Deaf, which subsequently succeeded in establishing St. Mary's School for Deaf Girls in Cabra, Dublin, with the help of the Dominican sisters in Cabra. Two of the nuns received training in Caen in the spirit of Abbé de l'Epée using sign language in order to educate deaf children with a minimal amount of speech. In 1846, the first year of the school's existence, 15 deaf girls were admitted (Figure 2.1 taken from Matthews 1996:64[9]).

This, however, did not accommodate the need for a school for deaf boys, which was established, after long negotiations, in 1849 in Dublin. The school was called St. Joseph's Prospect, Glasnevin, Dublin, and 35 boys were enrolled by 1851. However, the number of pupils increased rapidly, soon exceeding the number of pupils that could be accommodated on the grounds. In 1856, the Christian Brothers in Cabra took on the responsibility for the deaf school and St. Joseph's School for Deaf Boys was established in Cabra, Dublin. To date, St. Joseph's and St. Mary's remain the only national schools dedicated to deaf education in Ireland (Figure 2.2 is taken from Matthews 1996:66).

The strict segregation of boys and girls, who were also discouraged from mixing socially outside school (Le Master & Dwyer 1991), led to the development of distinct male and female varieties of ISL described in section 2.1. The ISL variety of the opposite sex had to be learnt after graduation or when signers started dating signers of the opposite sex. As gender variation is still a feature of present day ISL, this segregation had a profound

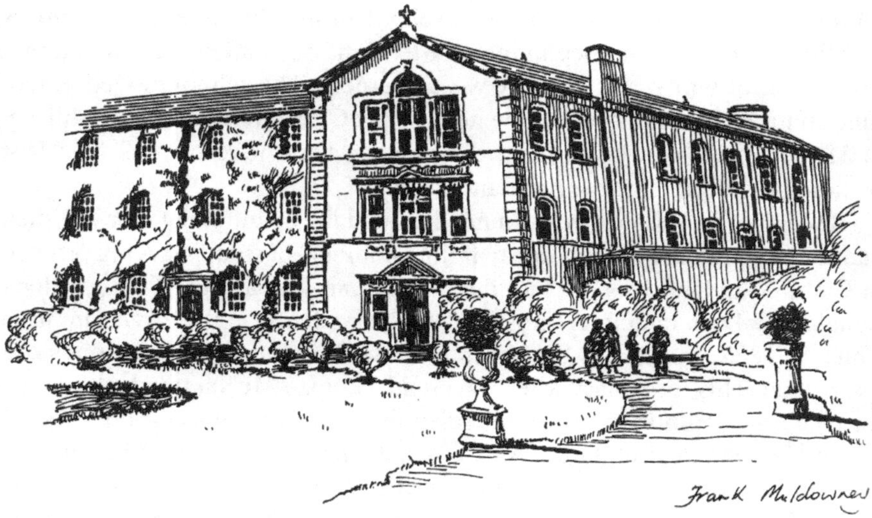

Figure 2.1 St. Mary's School for Deaf Girls, Cabra

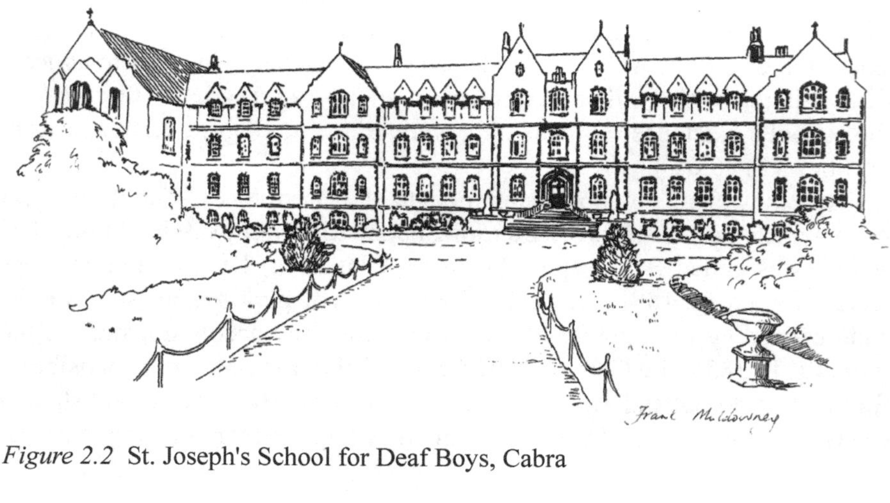

Figure 2.2 St. Joseph's School for Deaf Boys, Cabra

impact on the development of the language. Similar situations can also be found in other sign languages, such as LSQ, the sign language used in Québéc.

A final factor worth mentioning in the context of deaf education in Ireland is oralism, which was introduced to Ireland in the 20th century. Due to the Milan Congress in 1880[10], sign language was banned from schools across Europe and replaced by a wave of oral teaching methods using only spoken languages as medium of instruction. Oralism came to Ireland comparatively late. It was introduced to the Protestant school around 1918, to St. Mary's in 1946, and to St. Joseph's in 1957. It is essential that this time difference of 10 years between the girls' and the boys' schools be kept in mind as it will be crucial for the later analysis of mouthings. Today, the schools' current language policy states that teachers should communicate with the children in whatever language is most suitable to their needs, be it Irish Sign Language, Signed English or spoken English (D.E.S. Inspectors' Report 2004 for St. Mary's). Also, more and more children attend local, mainstream schools in partially deaf units as their parents refrain from sending them to a boarding school in Dublin or moving to the capital. This probably has a major impact on the language of these children, as they lack adult Deaf role models who competently use ISL. Instead, they might be more influenced by hearing adults and the English language.

As was shown here, many factors have influenced deaf education in Ireland since the 19th century. The most important ones are a strict segregation of deaf boys and girls at school which led to the development of distinct varieties of ISL, and the introduction of oralism to the two Dublin schools at different periods.

2.3. Structural Issues: The Use of Space

For communication, signed languages, as opposed to spoken languages, make use of the visual-gestural modality instead of the oral-aural modality. They especially use this different modality as well as space for their grammar in similar ways. Without a description of the use of space, it would be impossible to provide a full account of the grammar of a sign language (Keller 1998). In the following, some of the most important features linked to the visual-gestural modality and the use of space will be outlined.

Firstly, a few general issues should be mentioned. The most basic but also most important notion referring to the use of space in sign languages is that of the signing space. This is a particular space extending from the waist outwards

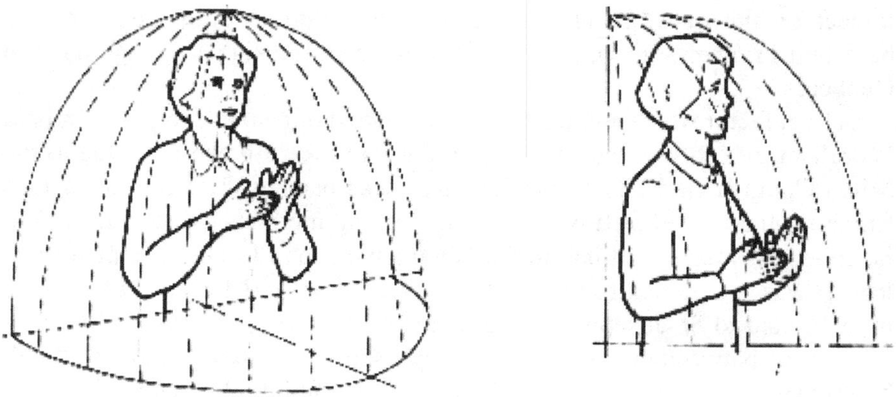

Figure 2.3 The signing space

and including the face and shoulders, in which all signs of a sign language have to be articulated (Ó Baoill & Matthews 2000). The signing space of ISL (taken from Ó Baoill & Matthews 2000:40[11]) is shown in figure 2.3.

All linguistic information is expressed visually in this signing space. In order to ensure grammatical clarity, this space is sub-divided as morphemes are articulated at given loci in relation to the signer or from the signer's perspective in pronominal reference, for example (Ó Baoill & Matthews 2000). Pronominal reference and verb agreement are discussed in more detail at the end of this section. Firstly and more generally, it should be mentioned that most lexical signs in Western sign languages are confined to the signing space. Its limits are dictated by ease of articulation and are only rarely exceeded.

The use of this sign space was claimed to be a universal feature of all signed languages in the world. The study of shared sign languages that are completely different from most European urban sign languages, however, has revealed that they make very different use of space. "Shared" sign languages (Nyst 2012) are found throughout the whole world and are usually confined to small speech communities, often in agricultural communities or fishing towns (Nonaka 2004). As opposed to the sign languages of the Western hemisphere, which are mostly minority languages spoken by the deaf population of a country, these languages are shared, i.e. they are used by hearing and deaf people alike.[12] The signing space of these languages is much larger, some movements (like walking, for example) are acted out, and absolute spatial reference is used (Zeshan 2008).

Space is very important for all linguistic levels of sign languages. For instance, the location of a sign is a phonological parameter that can be meaning distinguishing in minimal pairs.[13] In the following, two phenomena related to the use of space in sign languages will be outlined: verb agreement and pronominal reference. Both are crucial for the investigation of the ISL data in chapters 5 and 6.

Traditionally, a tripartite classification of verbs is assumed for signed languages (Padden 1988). This distinction is based on Padden's (1988) study of ASL syntax. According to this classification, which is based on the spatio-morphological properties of sign language verbs, there are *plain verbs*, *spatial verbs* and *inflecting verbs*. Applying this distinction to other sign languages and other data sets, terminology varies considerably depending on different authors. The category of inflecting verbs has been re-named "directional verbs" (Prillwitz 1985) or "agreement verbs" (Liddel & Johnson 1987), while spatial verbs were re-named as "spatial-locative verbs" (Liddel & Johnson 1987). The literature on ISL refers to two main categories of verbs only: *morphologically unmarked* and *morphologically marked verbs* (Ó Baoill & Matthews 2000). Other researchers have questioned a tripartite division of sign language verbs on morphological grounds, categorizing it as a semantic classification (Keller 1998; Meir 2002). Nevertheless, in order to give a full account of the sign linguistic literature, the traditional tripartite division is described briefly below.

Plain verbs are not very relevant when analyzing the use of space in signed languages. They are defined as having a fixed or constant place of articulation in space and do not take agreement for person, for instance. Examples of this type of verb are LOVE or HATE in ISL (Ó Baoill & Matthews 2000:124).

In contrast to plain verbs, morphologically marked verbs use spatial loci in order to realize inflection for person. These spatial loci have already been mentioned in the context of the use of space in general. Spatial loci may either refer to loci associated with locative arguments (locative agreement) or to loci linked to certain referents of the discourse (subject and object agreement) (de Quadros & Quer 2008). The morphological realization of agreement is the movement between two points associated with the arguments of certain verbs (de Quadros & Quer 2008). The differentiation that is generally made between agreement verbs and spatial verbs refers to the different kinds of inflection (either inflecting for location or for certain referents) that are shown. However, this distinction is questioned by certain researchers (Keller 1998). In his study on the use of space in DGS, Keller found that there is no basic (morphological) difference between the referential loci of spatial verbs and the referential loci of agreement verbs.[14] This claim is in line with the literature on ISL arguing that the verb category is subdivided into two different classes only.

The movement of morphologically marked verbs may express inflection for person, objects, location and manner in ISL (Ó Baoill & Matthews 2000). Person and location agreement is expressed by movement between two pre-established loci in the signing space. Object inflection may also be realized in this way, or by the use of a handling classifier.[15] Manner inflections are usually expressed by a modification of the movement patterns of the citation form of a sign. WALKING-IN-A-STRAINED-MANNER, e.g., would require a slower movement pattern than simply WALKING. The literature on ISL has so far subsumed both categories of verb marking (spatial and agreement) under the heading of "deictic verbs" (Ó Baoill & Matthews 2000:126).

A typical example of an agreement verb in sign languages is the ditransitive verb *to give*. It also exemplifies the workings of person agreement in sign languages very well. A picture of the locations of singular person agreement for the ISL verb GIVE can be seen below (figure adapted from Prillwitz 1985).

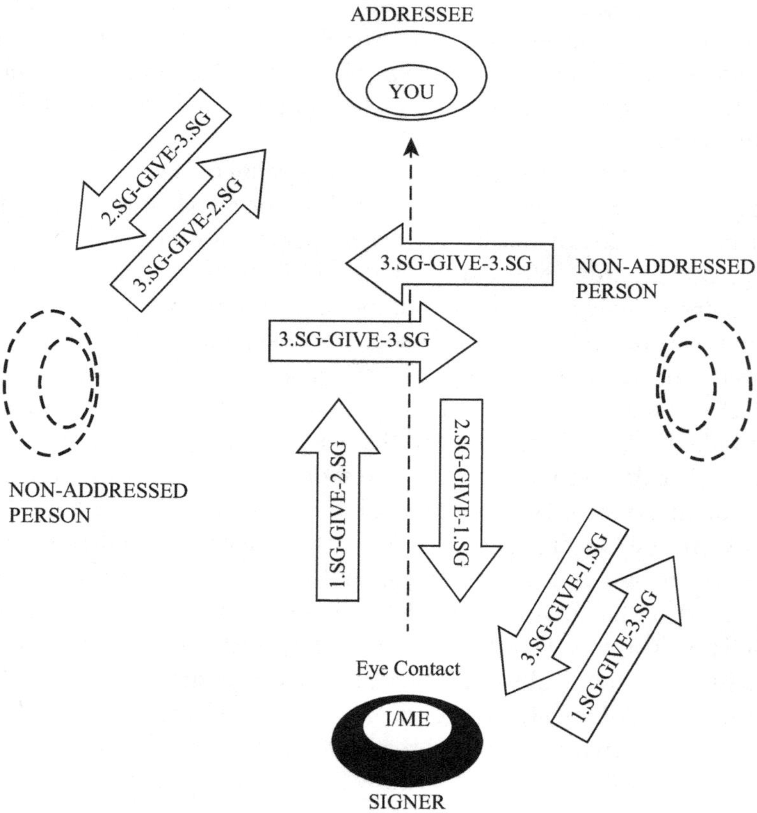

Figure 2.4 Locations of singular person agreement in the signing space

As can be seen in the picture above, the first person singular locus (I/ME) is in the bottom circle of the picture. The second person singular locus (ADDRESSED PERSON) is right in front of the signer. A third person singular locus (NON-ADDRESSED PERSON) might either be located to a signer's left or right. These locations are approximate and by no means absolute, especially referring to non-addressed participants. These might be located at any point that is not directly opposite the signer, which creates an ultimately infinite choice of locations for third person loci, a fact that has led to huge controversies between different sign linguists. This controversy is elaborated on in more detail in section 6.1.4.

Along with these conventionalized locations of personal pronouns in the signing space, the context of an utterance often determines the path of the movement of a verb. Sandler and Lillo-Martin (2006:479, f.) provide a good example of this from ASL:

> [...] Once a referent (say, Kim) has been associated with a location in space (say, on the right), then this pronoun [locus] will be used when a pronoun picks out a referent – in this case, by pointing towards the location associated with Kim on the right. Similarly, agreeing verbs taking Kim as an argument will move with respect to this location.

An interesting case is verbs that inflect for person, except for the first person singular as an object. This leads Ó Baoill and Matthews (2000) to call them "restricted verbs". Examples of this verb type are ASK and TELL. ASK in two different forms is depicted below (taken from Ó Baoill & Matthews 2000:135, f.).

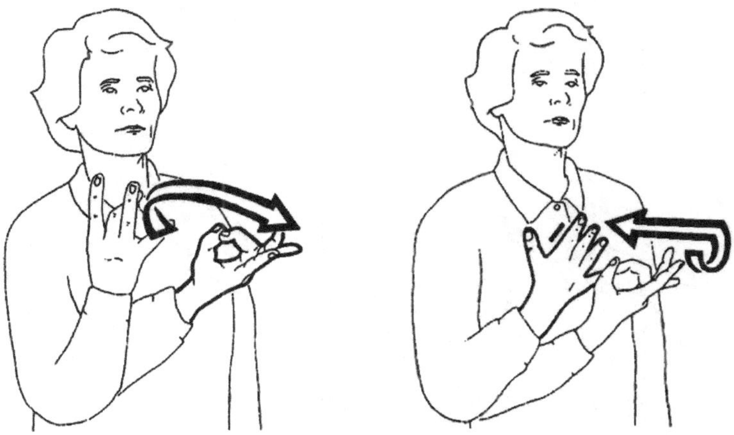

Figure 2.5 ISL sign ASK inflecting for person

As can be seen, in the second sentence the verb does not inflect for the 1SG object but expresses this periphrastically by using an index (ME). This is contrary to the first sentence in which the 2SG object is inflected on the verb by using the 2SG locus as the end point of the verb.

Ó Baoill and Matthews (2000) mention another interesting phenomenon in the context of morphologically marked verbs, namely items that would be considered predicative adjectives in English. They may function as predicates in ISL which is (similar to other sign languages) a copula-less language. They also seem to belong to the lexical class of verbs, however, this issue will be treated in detail in section 6.2. RIGHT and WRONG are examples of verbs that can inflect for person (Ó Baoill & Matthews 2000:138).

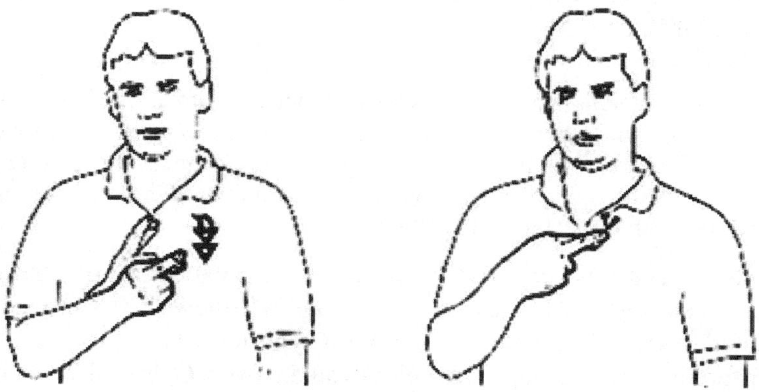

ISL PRO_2-RIGHT and PRO_1-RIGHT

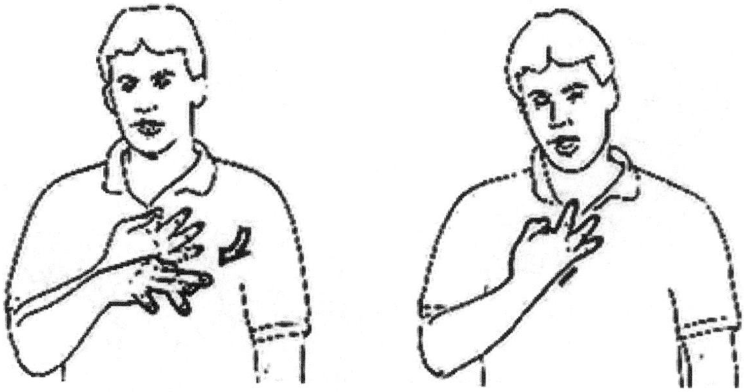

ISL PRO_2-WRONG and PRO_1-WRONG

Figure 2.6 Person inflections in ISL

This phenomenon seems to be restricted to certain signs of this kind as SICK in constructions like YOU (PRO_2) SICK cannot inflect for person (Ó Baoill & Matthews 2000:126).

Morphologically marked verbs may also inflect for a combination of person and number. This can be seen in the example of the ISL verb MOCK which would be reduplicated with a reversed direction of movement in order to express 'They mock me'. Below, the citation form of the sign MOCK is shown (Ó Baoill & Matthews 2000:128).

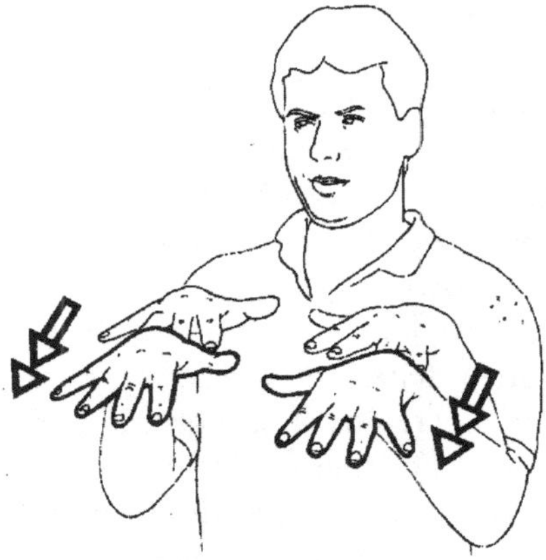

Figure 2.7 The ISL sign MOCK

Finally, a typical example of a verb of motion should be mentioned. This is the verb FLY shown below (Ó Baoill & Matthews 2000:145).

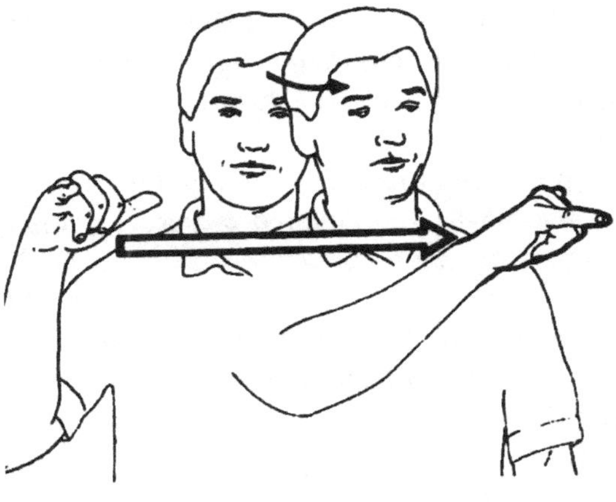

Figure 2.8 The ISL sign FLY

According to the distinction set up by Padden (1988) and made by many other researchers, this should be a completely different type of verb as compared to agreement verbs like GIVE. However, as previously mentioned, this distinction is not so much a morphological as a semantic one. While agreement verbs usually denote transfer in space, spatial verbs denote motion in space (Aronoff et al. 2005). In line with Ó Baoill and Matthews' (2000) account of the verb class in ISL, Padden's distinction is not considered applicable.

2.4. Structural Issues: Iconicity

Iconicity (generally referring either to the reflection of the extra-linguistic world in linguistic structures or the influence of human cognition on language) in sign languages has been a rather controversial topic ever since the beginnings of signed language research in the 1960s. The development of the formal linguistics framework at the time and during later decades, complicated research in the domain of motivatedness of signs considerably. Formal linguistic theories denied a link between language generation and cognition or extra-linguistic reality. Consequently, "proper" linguistic structures had to be arbitrary, which had already been a point in linguistics since its formulation in Saussure's lectures at the beginning of the 20th century (Saussure 1989). The issue of arbitrariness has been taken up very readily for theories of linguistic universals (e.g. Hockett 1960) and the like. However, the communication systems of the deaf around the world show a greater or more obvious amount of iconicity, especially on the lexical level, than spoken languages. It is thus not surprising that most studies on iconicity in sign languages tried to explain it away: Frishberg (1976) observed that iconicity diminishes in signs over time and Bellugi and Siple (1975) argued that it does not play a role for memorizing signs, as did Poizner et al. (1981), while Thompson et al. (2006) similarly showed that it is not decisive in "tip of the finger phenomena".

Recently, the importance of iconicity for sign linguistic systems has been emphasized. As iconicity was rediscovered as a crucial concept in functional approaches to linguistics, many researchers focused on iconicity in sign languages (Wilcox & Wilcox 1995, Pizzuto & Volterra 2000, Taub 2001, Pietrandrea 2002). Within the framework of cognitive linguistics or cognitive grammar as developed by Langacker (1991), Wilcox (2004) introduced the concept of cognitive iconicity as a special case of iconic motivation. He proposes that "the phonological and semantic poles of a symbolic structure reside in the same region of conceptual space". Other researchers have argued that the linguistic principle of arbitrariness has to be modified for sign languages and their different modality (Kutscher 2010), introducing new categories to the traditional semiotic model by Peirce, for instance. Van der Kooij (2002), Brentari (2007), Wilbur (2010) and Brentari (2012) have also stressed the importance of iconicity in sign phonology. For mouth actions in sign languages it is a rather important phenomenon, as will be discussed in relation to echo phonology in 3.2.2 and mouth gestures as ideophones in 6.2.4.

Further, it should be mentioned that mainly lexical iconicity was criticized and discussed controversially. Diagrammatical iconicity that is also observed in spoken language structures such as serial verb constructions, e.g. (cf. also Nanny & Fischer 1999), were not picked up as a topic in the controversy. The feature of lexical iconicity contributes in a unique way to similarities between sign languages around the world, resulting in higher mutual intelligibility between all languages of a supposed sign language family (Guerra Curie et al. 2002; Russo 2005). Lexical similarity is higher in sign languages than in spoken languages (Wilkinson 2009) which is due to a "shared symbolism" after Guerra Curie et al. (2002). Many studies have investigated this issue, hence Kyle and Woll (1985) compared approximately 250 lexical items from 15 sign languages and found a lexical overlap of 35–40%. It is now an undisputable fact that sign languages exploit iconicity as extremely productive constructions since the visual modality is especially well suited for this.

It should be mentioned, however, that despite the view expressed by some researchers in the field (Sandler & Lillo-Martin 2006), iconicity is not self-evident but interpreted on the basis of the language user's perception of the construal between a sign and its referent. This means that signs are by no means transparent and thus easily understood by people outside the speech community. Supporting this statement, Adam et al. (2007) conducted a study for which signers of different nationalities had to judge the iconicity of signs. They report that signers perceived their own signs to be more iconic than the foreign signs. In Mohr (2007) I conducted a study on the transparency of DGS signs. In a sub-study, another test with native speakers of DGS was conducted in order to determine the degree of iconicity and transparency of ASL signs. The foreign language signs were not perceived as iconic and were not transparent.

From the results obtained in the studies described above, it has become clear that despite the high degree of lexical iconicity that can be observed in all sign languages around the world, this phenomenon is strongly culturally determined and does by no means lead to completely identical sign languages worldwide. The choice of a sign's iconic feature is arbitrary which adds to the arbitrary face of the sign: Wilkinson (2009) also states that arbitrariness and iconicity are not mutually exclusive but are both realized in a sign. This mechanism might be compared to occurrences of onomatopoeia in spoken languages that are language and culture specific, although all are iconic in their own way.

Naturally, the lexicon of ISL also contains items that can be perceived as being iconic, such as DRINK, TELEPHONE or KEY. The sign KEY is depicted below (taken from Ó Baoill & Matthews 2000:145).

Apart from iconicity on the lexical level, iconic constructions can be found in morphosyntax. Having outlined the mechanisms of verb marking in section 2.3, another phenomenon shall be mentioned in the context of iconicity. Besides inflecting for person (subject), ditransitive verbs like GIVE also show object agreement. Thus, the picture below shows the ISL sentence PRO$_1$-GIVE-CYLINDRICAL-OBJECT (glass)-PRO$_2$ meaning 'I give a glass to you' (taken from Ó Baoill & Matthews 2000:127).

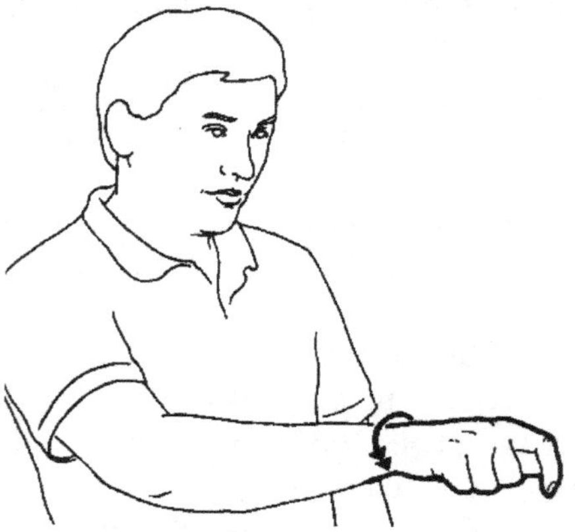

Figure 2.9 The ISL sign KEY

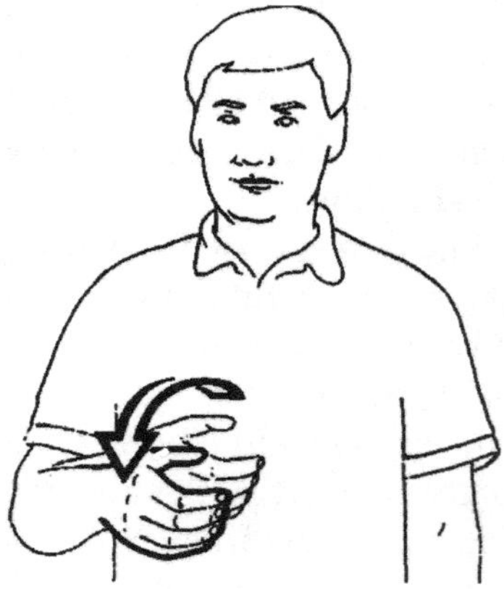

Figure 2.10 ISL: PRO$_1$-GIVE-CYLINDRICAL-OBJECT (glass)-PRO$_2$

In the above sentence, a classifier handshape is used. In this case, it is the classifier for cylindrical objects. If the signer gave another object, like a piece of paper, to the interlocutor, the classifier for a flat, thin object would be used. The type of handling classifier which is relevant for examples such as figure 2.10 represents the shape of a hand or any other object handling or gripping the referent. The iconic character of the classifier is clearly evident in examples like these. Classifier constructions in general, as well as in the context of iconicity, are a rather controversial topic in sign linguistics. In the early days of sign linguistics they were considered to be "mimetic" and "pantomime" (e.g. Klima & Bellugi 1979) and hence rather neglected by researchers in the field. Consequently, they were only accredited very late in the literature. The first systematic analysis of their properties (in ASL) was conducted by Supalla (1982; 1986). His original categorization mentioned Size and Shape Specifiers (SASSes) and semantic classifiers which are sometimes referred to as entity classifiers for ASL (Sandler & Lillo-Martin 2006). A third type of classifier has been introduced, namely handling classifiers (cf. Figure 2.10). However, other categorizations of classifiers exist. Hence, Meir (2001) postulates theme and instrumental classifiers.

Generally, classifiers in sign languages are "complex predicates in which movement, handshape, and location are meaningful elements" (Brentari 2012). This is in line with Ó Baoill and Matthews (2000), who mention that classifiers in ISL are largely used predicatively while they are mostly used in arguments in spoken languages. Despite the fact that classifiers are attested for all European and North American (urban) sign languages and show striking similarities concerning their form, function and use, there are cross-linguistic differences with respect to the inventory of classifiers. For ISL, Ó Baoill and Matthews (2000) mention that classifiers can be subdivided into two major categories, namely classifiers for animate and inanimate entities.

Benedicto and Brentari (2004) and Brentari (2012) make another interesting claim about the iconicity of classifier constructions. Referring to Engberg-Pedersen's four-way distinction of classifiers, i.e. whole entity, surface, limb/body part, handling, they found that only limb/body part and handling classifiers can use orientation in a morphological way (changing the orientation of a handling classifier is grammatical while changing it in a surface classifier is not). An even distribution of the expression of orientation across classifier types would be more iconic according to them (Brentari 2012:44) but grammar functions as a constraining factor in this case.

After this short outline of iconicity in sign languages, we will now turn to simultaneous constructions. These are described briefly in the following section.

2.5. Structural Issues: Simultaneity

In spoken languages, most linguistic material is ordered sequentially, i.e. morphemes are put in strings in order to convey meaning, phonemes form strings to form morphemes. The only areas in spoken languages in which information is ordered simultaneously are intonation and prosody. Here, the stress of a word, voice pitch or different intonational contours are uttered simultaneously with a syllable, a word or a sentence. In sign languages, unique simultaneous constructions can be observed, due to the different modality they use. Sign phonology largely operates simultaneously, which is represented in several different phonological models (e.g. Stokoe 1960; van der Hulst 1993; Brentari 1998).[16] Moreover, sign language morphology can be analyzed as using simultaneous constructions (e.g. Klima & Bellugi 1979; Zwitserlood 2003; Schwager 2004; Aronoff et al. 2005; Schuit 2007). Finally, the use of non-manual features often results in simultaneous constructions. As this phenomenon is discussed in detail in chapter 3, I will focus on a few examples of simultaneous phonological and morphological structures here.

Stokoe (1960) was the first to acknowledge that the signs of ASL are not holistic entities but rather consist of a relatively small number of meaningless units that can be combined to form meaningful signs. In his cheremic model, he showed that the features of handshape, location and movement are meaning-distinguishing and minimal pairs can be found. Besides these three parameters, two more features are now usually included in the list of meaning-distinguishing features in sign languages. Those are non-manual features and hand/palm orientation. As the sub-lexical structure of non-manuals has not been worked out sufficiently in any sign phonological model (Brentari 2012) and their uses and functions are discussed at length in chapter 3, they are not outlined here.[17] The inclusion of orientation as an independent parameter in sign phonology was proposed by Battison (1978). It remains controversial as there are only very few minimal pairs distinguished by orientation which is why several phonological models include it as a derivable feature (cf. e.g. Crasborn & van der Kooij 1997; Sandler & Lillo-Martin 2006; Brentari 2012). All distinguishing features, i.e. handshape, location, movement, orientation (and non-manual features) are combined simultaneously in order to form a sign. Thus, the hand has a certain handshape which has a certain orientation. The hand is moved from a certain location to another one, while the whole action is accompanied by certain non-manual features in most cases.

After the short outline of simultaneous processes in sign phonology, I will now turn to simultaneous morphology in sign languages. Several issues of simultaneous or non-concatenative morphology were tackled in the previous section already. Hence, it was shown that verbs in ISL can inflect for person, object, location and manner. This agreement is usually realized as a simultaneous morphological process which results in polycomponential signs. These constructions present a serious difficulty with respect to the linguistic description of the items. Phonology and morphology are not easily distinguished in these forms, just as morpheme boundaries cannot easily be identified. This is perhaps one of the reasons why sign morphology remains an under-researched topic.

An issue to be mentioned in the context of non-concatenative morphology in sign languages is aktionsart.[18] This will be highly important for the distinction of different word classes in ISL in chapter 6. As a simultaneous feature, in ASL certain aktionsart morphology changes the straight movement path of a verb to a circular movement (Klima & Bellugi 1979; Sandler 2003). In ISL, aktionsart marking is usually indicated sequentially by movement repetition, role-shifting, the completion marker, the accomplishment marker, the about-to marker or the left to right time line. Non-manual features constitute the only exception (Ó Baoill & Matthews 2000).[19]

It also seems noteworthy that the simultaneous affixation of an "aspect morpheme" or rather the general existence of simultaneous morphology is not restricted to sign languages only. Several phenomena found in tone languages are consequently analyzed as suprasegmental affixes that e.g. have aspectual value (Gilley 2004). Two examples (taken from Gilley 2004:5) from an African tonal language of the Nilotic branch of the Nilo-Saharan language phylum are given in (1) and (2).

(1) *ānéy ùcwòttɔ* *kī* *dhánhɔ* [Shilluk]
Aney NE:IMP:BEN-call IND person
'Someone is calling a person for Aney.'

(2) *ānéy ùc'wòttɔ* *kī* *dhánhɔ* [Shilluk]
Aney NE:PF:BEN-call IND person
'Someone called a person for Aney.'

As can be seen, the tone change from a low level tone to a high level tone causes a change from imperfective to perfective aspect. The morphological process that is used in this case is apparently also a simultaneous one.

Before concluding this section, I want to turn to a very unique morphological feature of sign languages that is due to the different modality as compared to spoken languages. In ISL, simultaneous compounds can be formed from two free morphemes. These formations are most comparable to blends in spoken languages in which two free morphemes "blend" into a new monomorphemic word from which neither the first nor the second morpheme is distinguishable. An example of this is the English word *smog*, formed from *smoke* and *fog*. In ISL, the combination of the signs TELEPHONE (with the normal place of articulation next to the signer's head) and TYPING (which is normally a double-handed sign) results in the compound MINICOM. The sign is shown below (taken from Ó Baoill & Matthews 2000:245).

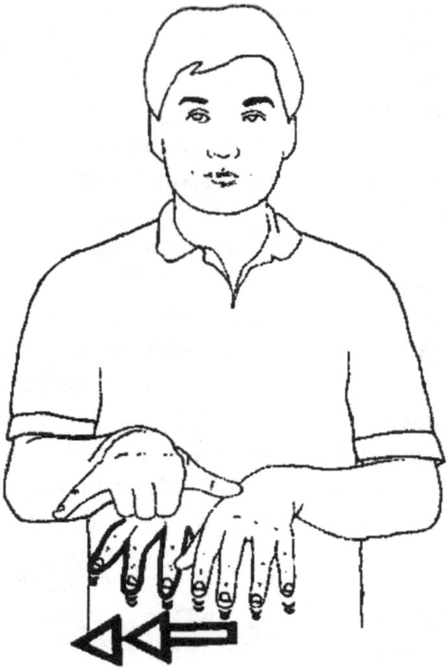

Figure 2.11 The ISL sign MINICOM

The difference between formations like these and blends from spoken languages is probably that both free morphemes are still distinguishable in the sign whereas they are not in a blend. As is apparent, the possibility of a formation like this derives from the use of the visual-gestural modality.

2.6. Structural issues: Non-manual Features

All sign languages of the world use non-manual features beside purely manual signs. Thus, ISL also uses certain non-manual features on different linguistic levels. This section will provide a brief overview of the non-manual features used in ISL. While mouth actions form an integral part of non-manuals, they are discussed in detail in chapters 5 and 6. Only a few examples will be mentioned in the current section.

The non-manual features mentioned by Ó Baoill and Matthews (2000) are: eyebrow movement, movement of the eyes, mouth patterns, blowing of the cheeks, tilting of the head and shoulder movements. They mention that non-manuals are especially used in order to express syntactic relations or lexical distinctions. Moreover, certain morphological functions such as the marking of the comparative and superlative by adding certain facial expressions to the manual sign are noted. An example of a comparative can be seen in the example of COLD - COLDER in figure 2.12 (taken from Ó Baoill & Matthews 2000:179).

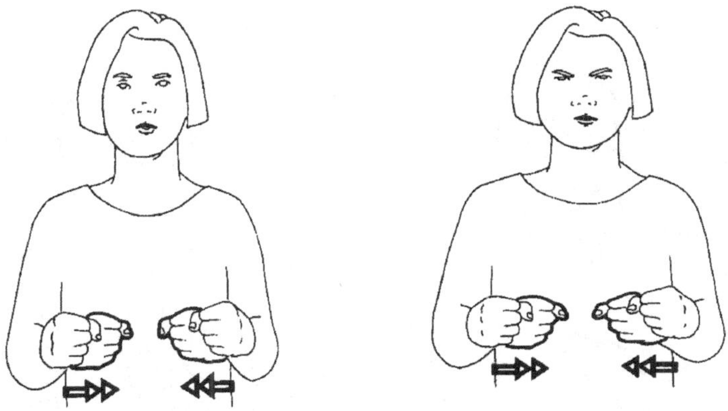

Figure 2.12 The ISL sign COLD and COLDER

On the phonological level, non-manual features serve to distinguish minimal pairs. Thus, a change in facial expression distinguishes the signs DISBELIEF/WARY/UNSURE on the one hand and FALSE on the other (Ó Baoill & Matthews 2000:50).

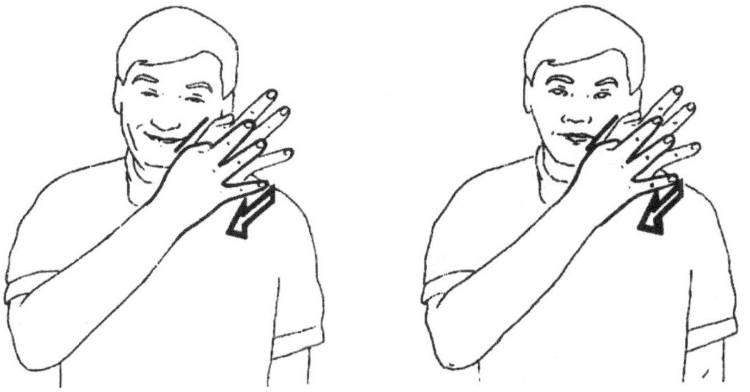

Figure 2.13 The ISL signs DISBELIEF/WARY/UNSURE and FALSE

Besides examples such as those mentioned above, a sign may acquire a different meaning by adding different non-manual features (especially facial expressions). In this case, the non-manual feature is not an inherent formational feature of the sign itself but rather a pragmatic means comparable to the use of suprasegmentals and especially intonation in spoken languages. An example of this can be seen below. The pictures show the manual sign WHO accompanied by different non-manual features and thus meaning 'Who?', 'Who!' and 'You are not who I think you are, are you!' (taken from Ó Baoill & Matthews 2000:174). The last sign is also accompanied by a side-to-side headshake.

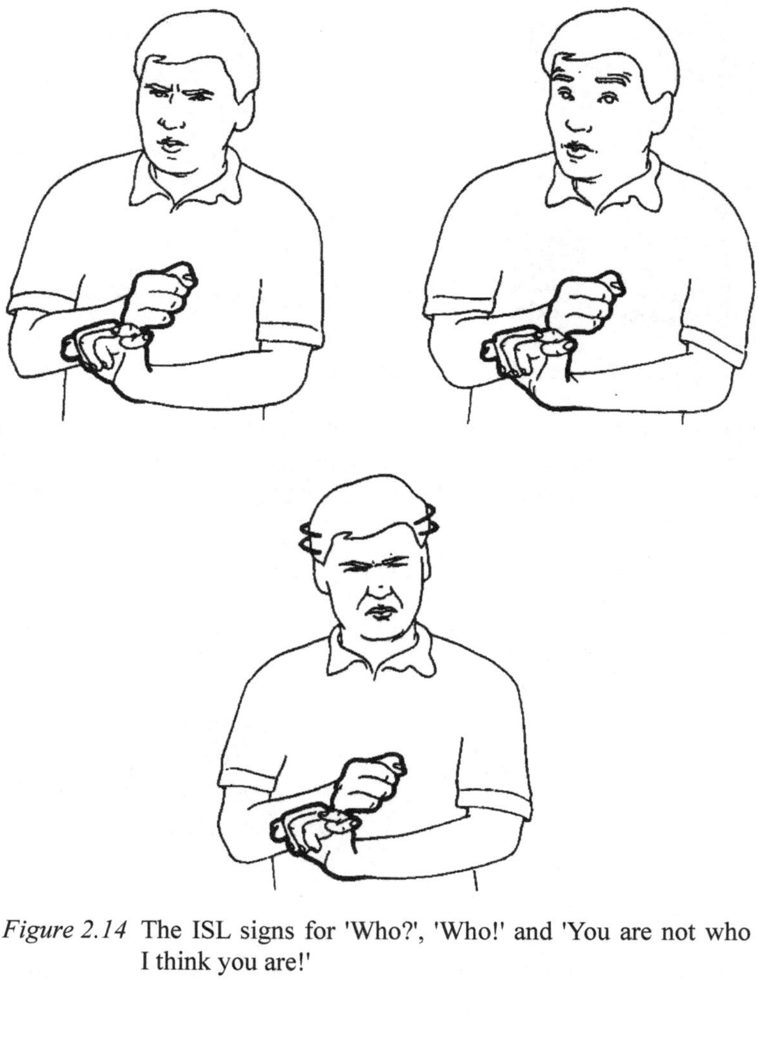

Figure 2.14 The ISL signs for 'Who?', 'Who!' and 'You are not who I think you are!'

Moreover, non-manuals may also serve to fulfill adverbial function when combined with verbs. Ó Baoill and Matthews (2000:180) mention five manners or degrees of actions that are often expressed in ISL:

1. Degree of difficulty
2. (Objects being handled are) Thin and delicate
3. (Action performed) With clumsiness
4. Relaxed manner
5. Non-existence of a previous existing entity

An example of "degree of difficulty", (Ó Baoill and Matthews 2000:180) can be seen in figure 2.15 below.

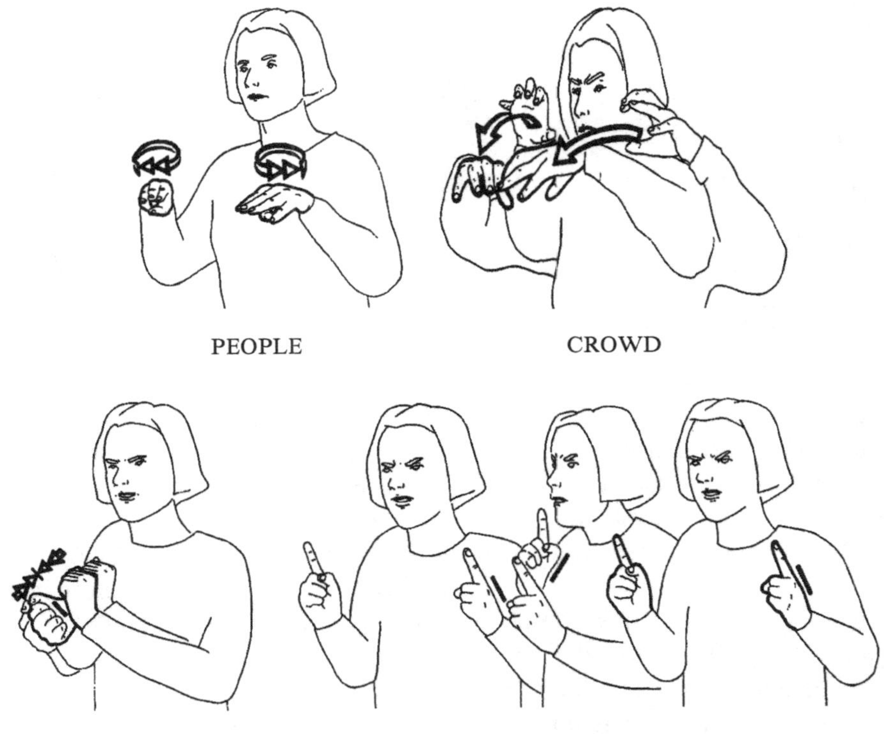

Figure 2.15 'It was difficult to get through the crowd.'

In this case, the non-manual marker accompanying ME-MOVE-THROUGH-THEM expresses "degree of difficulty". This emphasizes the fact that non-manual markers which look very similar (e.g. furrowed brows seen in several of the previous pictures), operate on different linguistic levels, serve different linguistic functions and modify meanings in different ways.

Finally, turning to the syntactic level, non-manual features are important for question formation, topic-comment structures and conditional sentences in ISL. Facial expression is often the only distinguishing feature between declarative sentences, questions and negations. More precisely, the non-manual features accompanying WH-questions in ISL are a forward tilt of the head and a slight downward movement, a lowering of the eyebrows and a narrowing of the eyes (Ó Baoill & Matthews 2000). This can be seen in the pictures of WHO, WHEN and WHERE below (taken from Ó Baoill & Matthews 2000:182).

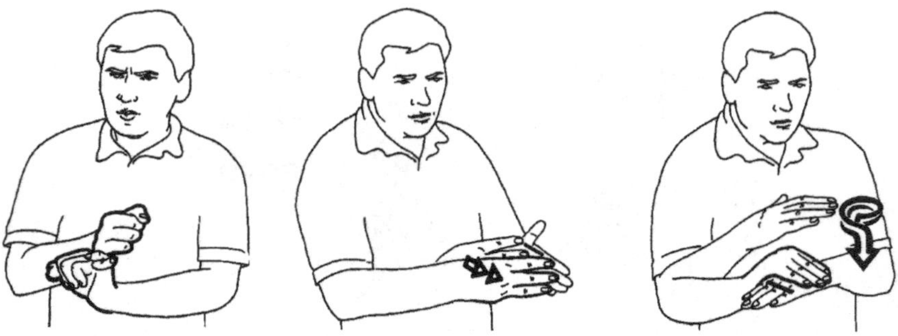

Figure 2.16 The ISL signs WHO, WHEN and WHERE

This is in line with findings from other sign languages and indeed substantiates Pfau and Quer's (2010) claim that lowered eyebrows usually accompany WH-constructions in the world's sign languages. The only difference is that Pfau and Quer mention a backward head tilt accompanying most WH-constructions while in ISL a forward head tilt is used.

Yes/no questions are accompanied by raised eyebrows, wide eyes and a forward movement of the head (Ó Baoill & Matthews 2000) which reflects cross-linguistic tendencies for this sentence structure mentioned by Pfau and Quer (2010). In ISL, too, the word order of a declarative sentence is kept, the non-manual features are thus the only indication of a question.

As far as negation is concerned, ISL forms part of the group of sign languages that might use a non-manual feature without using a manual negation particle in order to negate a sentence. In ISL, a side-to-side headshake is used in order to negate a sentence. However, negation particles such as NO, NEVER, NOTHING, etc. may be used as well. Thus, the sentence 'I do not understand' could be expressed in two different ways displayed in the examples below (both taken from Ó Baoill & Matthews 2000:186).

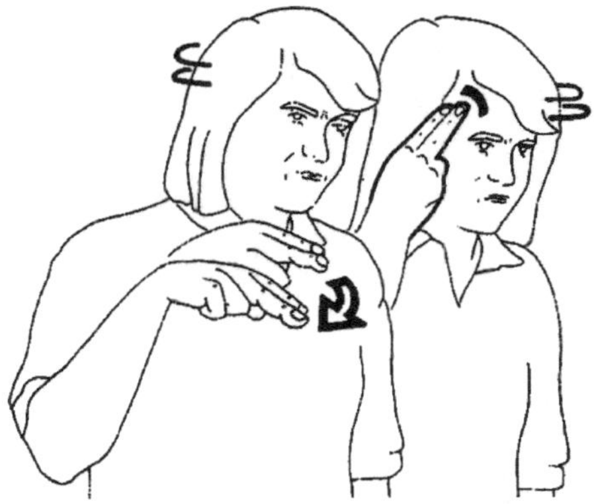

Figure 2.17 ISL for 'I don't understand' including a negation particle

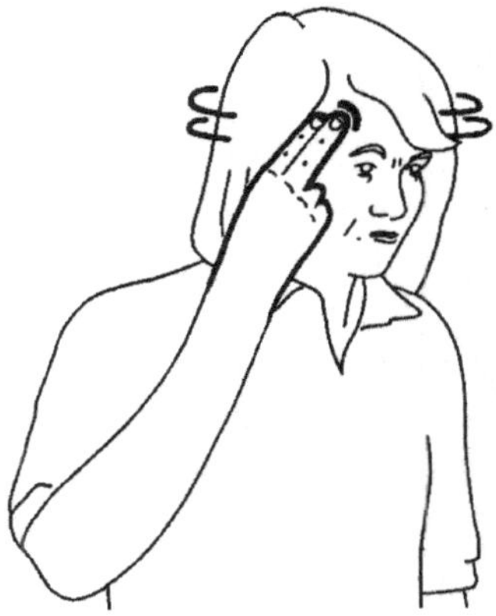

Figure 2.18 ISL for 'I don't understand' without a negation particle

The signer in figure 2.17 shows the negation of the sign UNDERSTAND including a negative particle (NOT) while the signer in figure 2.18 uses the side-to-side headshake only.

Topic-comment structures are very common in present-day ISL which is in line with the claim that sign languages are topic-prominent languages, such as Chinese, for example (cf. chapter 3.2.2). While there is no universally accepted definition of the term "topic", most definitions mention topics as the "sentence subject"[20] and comments as the "predicate" (Bußmann 2002).[21] One of the tests that can be applied in order to identify the topic of a sentence is asking the question "What about X?" (Gundel 1977). A topic provides the answer to this question.

The main non-manual features that are used in order to mark these constructions in ISL are a slight backward tilt of the head, raised eyebrows accompanying the topic and a slight headnod afterwards (Ó Baoill & Matthews 2000). An example of a topic-comment structure can be seen in the sentence 'That camera is mine' below (taken from Ó Baoill & Matthews 2000:188).

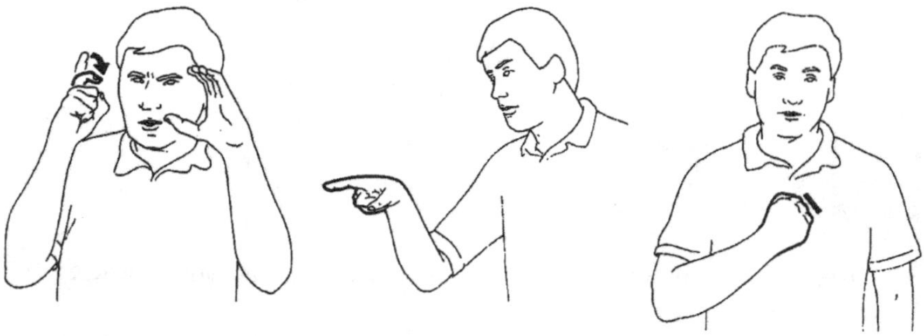

Figure 2.19 CAMERCA INDEX MINE - 'That camera is mine'

The transition from lowered to relaxed eyebrows between the topic (CAMERA) and the comment (MINE) is obvious in this example. Leeson and Grehan (2004) empirically researched topic-comment constructions in ISL and found that female signers often omit the tilting of the head used to mark a topic. This shows that gender differences permeate the lexical level in ISL. Moreover, they found that some signers use eye blinks to mark the offset of a topic. This, however, seems not to be obligatory.

Finally, conditional clauses are marked in a way similar to that of topic comment constructions. Ó Baoill and Matthews (2000) mention a raising of the head, raised eyebrows and wide open eyes as the non-manual features used to mark conditionals. Moreover, they observed that in case a negative 'if' is involved or some doubt is attached to the conditional, the sentence is usually accompanied by a squint. This is similar to the findings of Dachkovsky and Sandler (2007) for Israeli Sign Language (IsSL)[22] discussed in chapter 3.2.2.

As was shown in this section, non-manual features are commonly used in ISL for different linguistic functions. On the phonological level, for instance, they distinguish minimal pairs. Further, they are also used for some morphological and various syntactical functions. A few differences between male and female non-manuals, such as the omission of the head-tilt as a topic marker in women, were also mentioned here. The use of mouth actions was rarely mentioned as it has not been systematically researched so far. Thus, chapters 5 and 6 will provide some insight into the system of mouth actions in ISL. The analysis in chapter 5 will especially shed some light on gender differences concerning non-manuals.

Chapter 3
Non-manuals in Sign Languages – Theoretical Background

Although it is a common belief that sign languages use the hands instead of the mouth for communication, this is only partly true. Pfau and Quer (2010) call this "one of the common misconceptions about sign languages". An expanding body of research on the various functions of non-manual markers in different sign languages since the 1980s (e.g. Coulter 1979; Woll 1981; Engberg-Pedersen 1990; Sandler 1999; Sutton-Spence & Woll 2006; Pfau & Quer 2010) has proven this statement to be wrong. Apart from the hands, other articulators such as the body, the head and different parts of the face are equally important for sign language communication. Thus, linguistically significant elements which are expressed by any articulator other than the hands are called "non-manual markers" or "non-manuals" (Pfau & Quer 2010). These non-manual markers encode various kinds of grammatical information as well as prosodic features such as intonation (Sandler & Lillo-Martin 2006; Sandler 2012). These grammatical non-manuals have to be distinguished from purely affective non-manual markers such as brow raises for surprise. These affective non-manuals are not the subject of this chapter. In figure 3.1 below, the hierarchy of grammatical non-manuals after Woll (2001:88) can be seen.

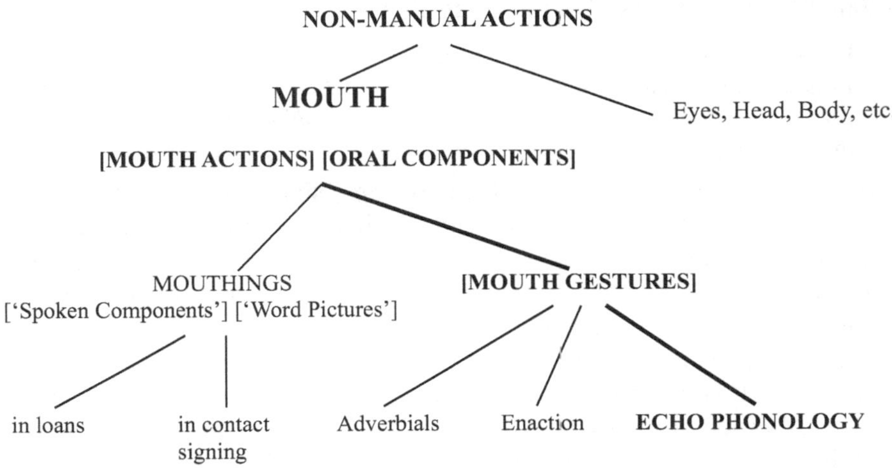

Figure 3.1 Hierarchy of non-manuals

As shown in Figure 3.1, non-manuals can generally be distinguished into those produced by articulators such as the eyes, the head or the body. These are thus not related to actions performed by the mouth. In the following, both types will be described concerning their function(s). While the first part of the chapter elaborates on non-mouth related actions by the eyes (3.1.1), the face (3.1.2 and 3.1.3), the second part (3.2) discusses mouth actions which are the focus of this book.

3.1. Non-Mouth Related Non-Manuals

As mentioned in 3, the current subchapter discusses the functions, i.e. grammatical, lexical and prosodic roles of non-manual markers produced by articulators other than the mouth. These are eye gaze, facial expression and its functions on the lexical, syntactic and prosodic level, and finally head movements such as headnods or headshakes. In line with Sandler (2012), non-manuals are not seen as a coherent linguistic category but as operating on different (linguistic) levels, be they prosodic, syntactic, lexical or pragmatic.

3.1.1. Eye Gaze

Eye gaze in sign languages has many important functions on several linguistic levels. As opposed to most of the other non-manuals, it does not fulfill prosodic functions, however (Sandler 2012). Sutton-Spence & Woll (2006:94) report at least five functions of eye gaze in BSL:

> [...] at the phonological level for lexical distinctions; in conjunction with the location and movement of referents in space; to show 'role shift'; to contrast pseudo-questions (rhetorical and echo) with genuine questions; and for marking time.

Concerning lexical distinctions, there are some signs, in which eye gaze is obligatory, e.g. BSL GOD and HEAVEN. Without the required eye gaze, the sign acquires a different or no meaning. An example of eye gaze fulfilling a meaning distinguishing function is the BSL signs GOD and BOSS below (from Sutton-Spence & Woll 2006:94[23]).

In cases like these, eye gaze is an essential part of the sign's phonological description. It serves to distinguish the minimal pair depicted in the above figure. Other non-manual features may have the same function, as will be shown in subsequent sections of this chapter. This emphasizes the importance of the inclusion of non-manuals in phonological models of the sign (cf. chapter 2.5).

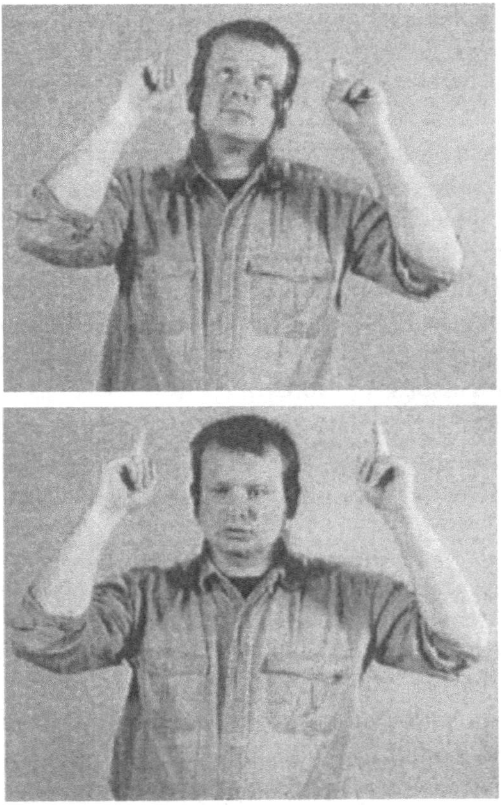

Figure 3.2 The BSL signs GOD and BOSS

Observing the morphological level, it has recently been argued that verb agreement can be expressed non-manually using eye gaze (Neidle et al. 2000; Pfau & Quer 2010). Thus, in transitive sentences a head tilt towards the subject[24] may express subject agreement while eye gaze towards the object may indicate object agreement. This is supposed to hold true for morphologically marked and morphologically unmarked verbs alike. An example can be seen in (1) (taken from Pfau & Quer 2010:393).

          ______head tilt-3a
          ______eye gaze-3b
(1) ANN$_{3a}$ $_{3a}$BLAME$_{3b}$ MARY$_{3b}$ [ASL]
'Ann blames Mary.'

However, Thompson et al. (2006) found that eye gaze accompanying morphologically marked verbs such as BLAME is often targeted towards the object, while in accompanying morphologically unmarked verbs such as LOVE it is often directed towards the addressee or some other location. It is thus not clear whether eye gaze can be used as a non-manual object marker with all kinds of verbs.

Finally, eye gaze (combined with head turns) has been argued to be used to distinguish different personal pronouns from each other. Hence, the direction of eye gaze, the degree of head turn and the direction of pointing align in second person pronouns (Pfau & Quer 2010). In third person pronouns however, these features are not aligned, as the eye gaze and the head follow the direction of the hand when pointing to the addressee. As the issue of pronominalization, especially referring to person distinctions, is still controversial in sign linguistics, more research in this area is needed to analyze unresolved issues.[25]

3.1.2. Facial Expression

In sign languages, facial expression is not exclusively used in order to express a speaker's emotions, although it is commonly used for this purpose by spoken and sign language users alike. It also fulfills many grammatical functions in sign languages with respect to several linguistic levels. It is a very complex linguistic feature that needs to take into consideration movements of the cheeks, brows and eyelids (Sutton-Spence & Woll 2006). Prillwitz (1985:63) even lists five constituents of facial expression:

1. Haltung von Kopf, Schultern und Oberkörper (Neigung, Schräge, Anspannung) (= 'position of the head, shoulders and torso (leaning, incline, tension)')
2. Augenbrauen (hochgezogen, zusammengezogen) (= 'eyebrows (raised, furrowed)')
3. Augenöffnung (weit geöffnet, zusammengekniffen, blinzeln) (= 'eye aperture (wide open, squint, blinking)')
4. Blickrichtung (geradeaus, zur Seite, nach oben/unten) (= 'direction of eye gaze (straight ahead, to side, upwards/downwards)')
5. Mundpartie (offen, geschlossen, zusammengepresst, Mundwinkel hoch- /runtergezogen, Kussmund, Unterlippe, Zunge) (= 'mouth (open, closed, pressed lips, corners up/down, puckered, lower lip, tongue)')

Although included in Prillwitz's list, body leans (1.) do not form part of facial expression, while eye gaze (4.) was already treated in chapter 3.1.1.

Actions of the mouth are discussed in detail in chapter 3.2. Hence, the relevant constituents to be described here are the eyebrows and eye aperture.

The interplay of different parts of facial expression in order to convey meaning is analyzed with respect to the lexicon/phonology, syntax and prosody or intonation where facial expression is crucial, too. Concerning the areas of syntax and intonation, it is controversial whether facial expression reflects either syntax or intonation. Thus, researchers such as Neidle et al. (2000) argue that grammatical facial expression is a direct reflection of syntax while researchers such as Wilbur (1991) and Sandler and Lillo-Martin (2006) do not agree with this theory and claim that facial expression corresponds to intonation. Trying to provide a balanced picture of the literature, both accounts will be discussed in the following.

3.1.2.1. Facial Expression and the Lexicon

One of the linguistic levels at which facial expression can be crucial for a sign is the phonological (lexical) level where it serves to distinguish signs from each other. In that case, facial expression is an essential part of the sign's phonological description (Pfau & Quer 2010:382) just like its handshape, orientation and other phonological parameters. However, facial expressions are not lexically specified for all signs, i.e. they are not obligatory for all manuals. Very often, facial expression is obligatory in signs assigning properties in the world's sign languages; examples of this would be HAPPY, SAD or RELIEVED. Here, the facial expression reflects the emotional state that is represented by the sign (Sutton-Spence & Woll 2006; Pfau & Quer 2010). Sutton-Spence and Woll (2006:88) suggest it is a mirror of emotion associated with meaning. Additionally, they mention that a particular facial expression associated with the meaning expressed by the sign (as in the case of HAPPY), can be superimposed on other signs or spread over the remainder of a sentence (Sutton-Spence & Woll 2006). They cite the BSL example SAD ME WHY RABBIT DIE in which the sad facial expression used in the sign SAD and spreading over the whole sentence would only be interrupted by the sign WHY which requires a special facial expression as a question marker (Sutton-Spence & Woll 2006:90f).

In some cases for which facial expression is lexically defined, a difference in facial expression may cause a minimal pair. Pfau and Quer mention an example from Catalan Sign Language (LSC) where the signs PITY and FALL-IN-LOVE are only distinguished by negative (furrowed brows and pursed lips) and positive facial expressions respectively (Pfau & Quer 2010:383[26]). The difference is visible in the figure below.

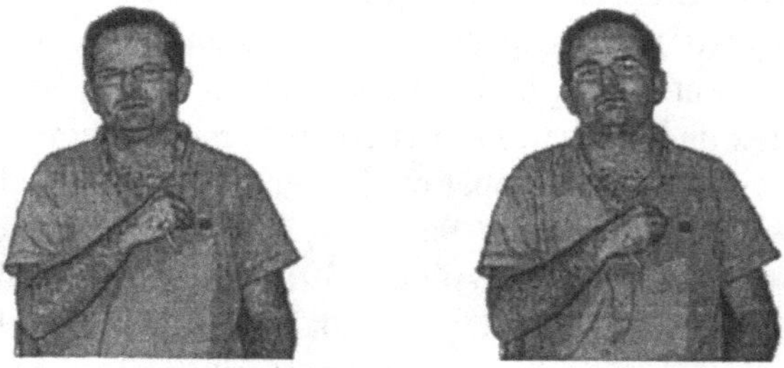

Figure 3.3 The LSC signs PITY and FALL-IN-LOVE

Finally, facial expression on its own, without being linked to any manual component, can be meaning-bearing. This is a common feature in all sign languages studied thus far, however, only certain (mostly property assigning or adverbial) meanings can be expressed by this means. Liddell (1980) already found that these are usually actions of the lower face. Pfau and Quer (2010:384f) mention the example of the diminutive and augmentative. Thus, in DGS a sucking in of the cheeks is associated with the diminutive and the blowing of one's cheeks with the augmentative. Pfau and Quer cite the following example for illustration[27]:

```
                         _____)(
(2)  POSS1 FRIEND HOUSE BUY                [DGS]
     'My friend bought a small house.'
```

As the meaning of this sentence is 'My friend bought a small house', the modifier 'small' is only expressed by the sucking in of the cheeks.

Furthermore, the same non-manuals may have adverbial function or serve as intensifiers when combined with the manual assigning the property. Hence, the sucking in of the cheeks combined with the manual SMALL would express the meaning 'very small' (Pfau & Quer 2010:385). Mouth actions fulfilling adverbial functions are discussed in section 3.2.1.

3.1.2.2. Facial Expression and Syntax

On the syntactical level, facial expression has been claimed to serve various functions. However, this was only discovered rather recently in sign language research leading to assumptions that sign languages have a very free sentence structure. This hypothesis seems logical, given that changes in word order as in topic-comment constructions, e.g., are marked by facial expression or other non-manual features. Thus, varying word orders were attributed to free sentence structures while the different construction types were not noticed. The importance of facial expression was simply not acknowledged.

The co-occurrence of certain facial expressions and syntactic constituents is discussed in the following section in which interrogation, topicalization, relative and conditional clauses are treated.

Firstly, a very general issue concerning facial expression and syntax should be mentioned. Facial expression can determine a sentence's meaning as far as statements, imperatives or negations are concerned. An example is the sentence WOMAN FORGET PURSE from ASL. The change of facial expression according to the meaning of the sign sequence can be seen below (taken from Liddell 1980[28]).

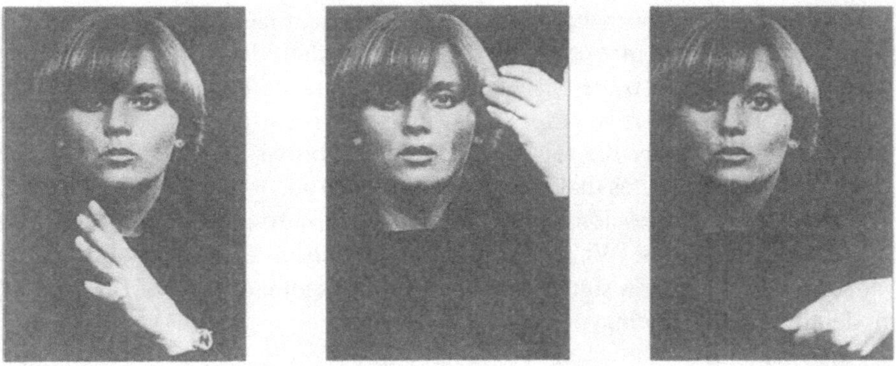

Figure 3.4 Grammatical facial expression in ASL - Statement

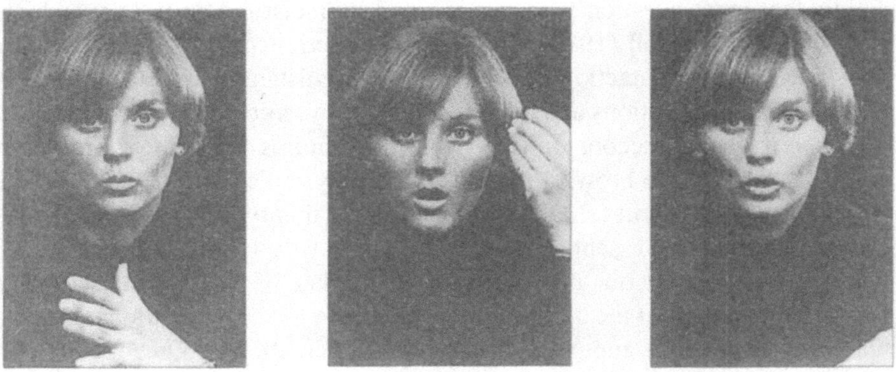

Figure 3.5 Grammatical facial expression in ASL - Question

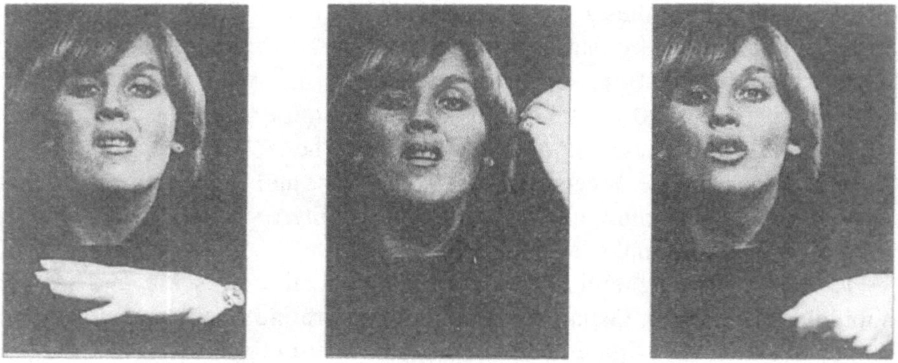

Figure 3.6 Grammatical facial expression in ASL - Relative clause

The first sequence of pictures (figure 3.4) is a mere statement 'The woman forgot the purse'. The second sequence (figure 3.5) is a question and the sign sequence is accompanied by several features of facial expression: raised brows and a forward movement of the head and shoulders. The last sequence of pictures (figure 3.6) represents the sign sequence being part of another sentence 'The woman who forgot the purse has just arrived'. The relative clause is indicated by the raised upper lip and brows and the tilting of the head. This demonstrates that just by changing the accompanying non-manual features (facial expression), one sign sequence may gain several different syntactical meanings. While the above was only a short overview of the existing possibilities in signed languages, some sentence types are discussed in detail in the following.

As was already shown above, facial expression is used in order to mark questions in sign languages. However, not all types of questions are marked by the same non-manual feature or even facial expression. Zeshan (2004) claims that most question types are marked by a distinct brow raise, which is in line with Liddell (1980) who states that actions of the upper face are usually related to syntactic functions. Cross-linguistically, differences occur between yes/no questions and WH-questions. In yes/no questions, the whole sentence is usually accompanied by raised eyebrows while the word order does not change, the brow raise is thus the only indication of the question (Dachkovsky & Sandler 2007). An example of this type of question is the above mentioned ASL sentence WOMAN FORGET PURSE (cf. figure 3.4). As was already pointed out, the non-manual marker of raised brows (and a forward movement of the head and shoulders) are the only question markers. Only very few sign languages (such as NGT, cf. Pfau & Quer 2010) use special (optional) question marking particles in order to mark a question.

WH-questions however, are usually accompanied by lowered eyebrows often combined with a slight backward head tilt (Pfau & Quer 2010). Differences in marking WH-questions occur cross-linguistically between languages where the facial expression accompanies the entire clause as in Italian Sign Language (LIS) (example 3), and languages like ASL where it is possible that facial expression is restricted to the WH-sign if it occurs sentence-finally (example 4, both from Pfau & Quer 2010).[29]

       ______________________________le
(3) TOMORROW HOUSE BUY WHO [LIS]
'Who will buy a house tomorrow?'

                                                    _____le
(4) TEACHER LIPREAD YESTERDAY WHO [ASL]
'Who did the teacher lipread yesterday?'

Examples like these have led for instance Neidle et al. (2000) to the conclusion that non-manual marking directly manifests syntactic structure (Sandler & Lillo-Martin 2006; Sandler 2012). According to them, the WH-question marker is determined by syntactical elements marked with the feature [+wh]. Their account of the obligatory spreading of the non-manual marker for in situ WH-elements is depicted below.

       _______________wh
(5) WHO LOVE JOHN [ASL]
'Who loves John?'

       __wh
(6) *WHO LOVE JOHN [+wh]$_C$ [ASL]

       ____________________wh
(7) *WHO LOVE JOHN[+wh]$_C$ [ASL]

In this case, there is no lexical material in the [+wh]$_C$ which is, suggest Neidle and colleagues, the reason for the obligatory spreading of the non-manual marker.

Another explanation for the non-manual WH-marker was put forward by Petronio and Lillo-Martin (1997). They claim that spreading of the non-manual marker is uniformly obligatory as according to them, the marker is a realization of the [+F, +WH] of the head C of an interrogative (Sandler &

Lillo-Martin 2006:451). This however, would contradict reality, as sentences such as (4) would be impossible. To them, these types of sentences are two sentence discourses with a null element. However, they admit that examples as in (8) (taken from Petronio and Lillo-Martin 1997:48) are more acceptable in clear discourse contexts.[30]

                                    _whq
(8) SOMEONE BUY CAR WHO [ASL]
'Someone bought a car. Who?'

A third account for the distribution is linked to intonation and prosodic constituents. However, syntactic and prosodic structures are closely linked so that it is not always easy to distinguish whether a certain feature should be attributed to syntax or intonation. Moreover, the relations between intonation and non-manual markers are elaborated on in section 3.1.2.3 and will thus not be treated further here. The only reported exception from the general pattern of WH-questions marked by lowered eyebrows, seems to be Indopakistani Sign Language (IPSL). Here, WH-questions are marked by raised eyebrows and a chin up and forward movement (Aboh et al. 2005 cited in Pfau & Quer 2010:388).

The next issue to be discussed is topics. While they are first and foremost concerned with information packaging serving a discourse function, and thus belong to the domain of pragmatics, topicalization also has an impact on the sentence structure which is why I treat topics in this section.

It is sometimes claimed that sign languages are topic-prominent languages such as Chinese. From a syntactic point of view, in sign languages just as in spoken languages, topics are usually realized by a constituent at the left edge of the sentence. While in spoken languages topics are often set apart from the remainder of the sentence by intonation, in sign languages they are accompanied by a non-manual marker. Pfau and Quer (2010:388f) mention that the basic marking for topics in sign languages is brow raise (as for example in Australian Sign Language (Auslan) and NGT) although it can be combined with other non-manuals depending on the information conveyed. For most sign languages, however, the subtle differences in layered non-manuals for topics have not been researched. For ASL however, topic markers have been clearly identified. Aarons (1994 as cited in Sandler and Lillo-Martin 2006:407) mentions three for ASL:

1. tm1: raised brows; head tilted slightly back and to the side; eyes widened; head moves down and forward

2. tm2: large movement of head back and to the side; eyes very wide, head moves down and forward
3. tm3: head forward, jerked slightly up and down; mouth open; upper lip raised, eyebrows raised; eyes wide open, fixed gaze, slight rapid headnods

The different topic markers are illustrated below (pictures taken from Sandler and Lillo-Martin 2006:408[31]):

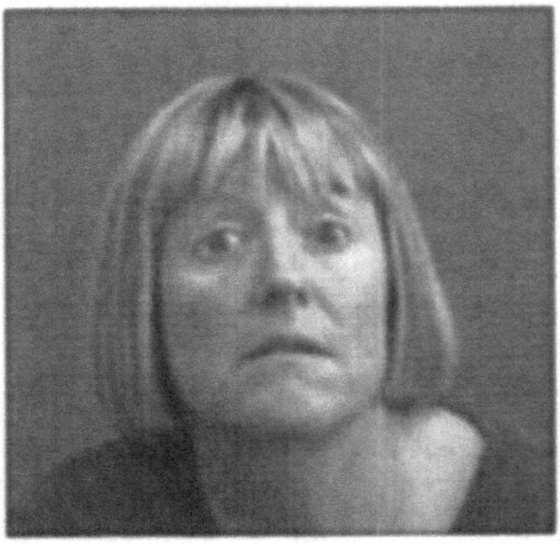

Figure 3.7 tm1 for ASL

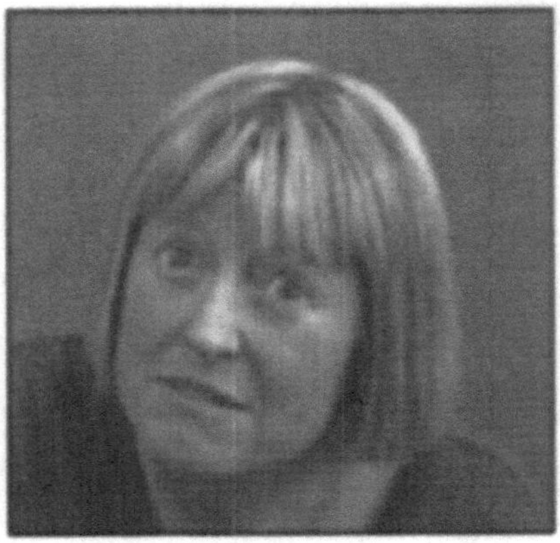

Figure 3.8 tm2 for ASL

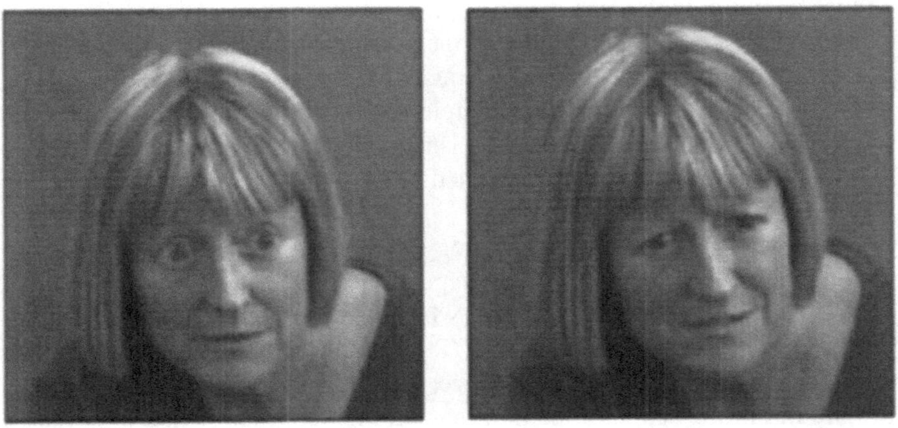

Figure 3.9 tm3 and alternative version for ASL

The choice of the different markers depends on the kind of topic and on the information conveyed. Sandler and Lillo-Martin (2006:407) define the different functions of tm1-3 as follows. Topics of the kind tm1 are used either to identify a particular member of the universe of discourse, for emphasis or for contrastive focus. Tm2 topics are employed in order to introduce new information which changes the discourse topic. Finally, tm3 topics could be translated by 'you know X'.

Additional concrete examples of differences between different topic markings can be cited for Hong Kong Sign Language (HKSL), where Sze's (2009:8) findings revealed that different kinds of topics such as scene-setting or aboutness topics are accompanied by different non-manuals such as brow-raising or head tilts. Moreover, non-manuals behave differently if sentences are negated or include a verb with a negative meaning.

(9) SECONDARY-TWO, START PLAY BASKETBALL, HAVE-COMPETITION, FARE-BETTER THAN [HKSL]
'At secondary two (=grade 8), I started playing basketball and had competitions; I was better than (other senior schoolmates).'

(10) LOUSY X-1 DISLIKE [HKSL]
'Lousy (handwriting), I don't like (it).'

While example (9) belongs to her group of scene-setting topics featuring an NP that sets up a temporal domain (Sze 2009:6) in which the topic is accompanied by a forward head tilt and raise, example (10) is called a "fronted non-grammatical object" which is normally not marked except in negations and when a verb with a negative meaning is involved.

For relative clauses, cross-linguistic tendencies can be identified as well. Thus, they are usually marked by raised eyebrows (Pfau & Quer 2010). This was already shown for the example WOMAN FORGET PURSE from ASL (figure 3.4). In this case, several non-manuals were layered as the relative clause was not only indicated by raised brows but also by a raised upper lip and tilting of the head.

However, there seem to be typology-related differences in the structure of relative clauses across sign languages. The use of head-internal relative clauses has been identified for ASL whereas the use of head-external relative clauses has been found in DGS (Pfau & Quer 2010; Pfau & Steinbach 2005 for DGS relative clauses). Hence, in DGS relative clauses, the head is usually out of the scope of the non-manual marker which either only marks the relative pronoun or extends over the whole relative clause.[32] This led Pfau and Steinbach (2005) to the conclusion that DGS relative clauses are externally headed. An example of this can be seen below (taken from Pfau & Quer 2010:393).[33]

_______re_(__)

(11) TOMORROW [MAN (INDEX$_{3a}$) [RPRO$_{3a}$ TIE BUY]] [DGS]
CONFERENCE GO-TO
'Tomorrow the man who is buying a tie is going to a conference.'

In languages such as ASL and LIS, the non-manual marker extends over the head noun as well. In LIS, the clause-final marker PE is added at the end of the relative clause. A typical relative clause construction in LIS would thus look like this (Pfau & Quer 2010:392):

______________________re

(12) [TODAY MAN$_3$ PIE BRING PE$_3$] YESTERDAY (INDEX$_3$) DANCE [LIS]
'The man that brought the pie today danced yesterday.'

As is obvious, the non-manual marker extends over the head noun MAN which is why these kinds of relative constructions are called head-internal.

Dachkovsky and Sandler (2007:26) found that in IsSL, relative clauses are usually marked by a squint. They argue that this is linked to a systematic correlation between the type of a linguistic construction, its pragmatic function and non-manuals. They claim that squints, e.g., are used when information has to be retrieved from the hearer's background knowledge.[34] Especially restrictive relative clause constructions were marked by a squint because the referent is "known or knowable to the addressee" (Dachkovsky & Sandler 2007:26) but not the current topic of the conversation. An example of this kind of construction can be seen below (Dachkovsky & Sandler 2007:26).

______________________________squint

(13) HOUSE INDEX$_1$ TOGETHER-WITH-YOU SEE INDEX RENT [IsSL]
'Finally we rented the apartment that I'd seen together with you.'

The function of the above relative clause is to move a referent that is not the centre of the current situation into that same centre of the communication. That is why a squint, which signals that the addressee has to retrieve some piece of information from his background knowledge, is used in this case. However, Dachkovsky and Sandler's investigation is one of the first systematic analyses of the correlations of pragmatic functions of sentence structures and non-manual features which remains to be done for other sign languages as yet.

Just like relative clauses, the non-manual marker for conditionals is the same cross-linguistically. Raised eyebrows are the most prominent feature and are usually combined with a raised chin, for instance. Usually, the clause that describes a hypothetical situation (= protasis) is accompanied by the non-manual feature. Also, it usually appears in sentence initial position (Pfau & Quer 2010:9).

Prillwitz (1985) provides an example of conditional clause marking in DGS. The conditional clause and the main clause are only distinguished by facial expression; no conjunctions are used. The transcription and the signed sentence are shown in figure 3.10 below (taken from Prillwitz 1985:57, drawing by Heiko Zienert):

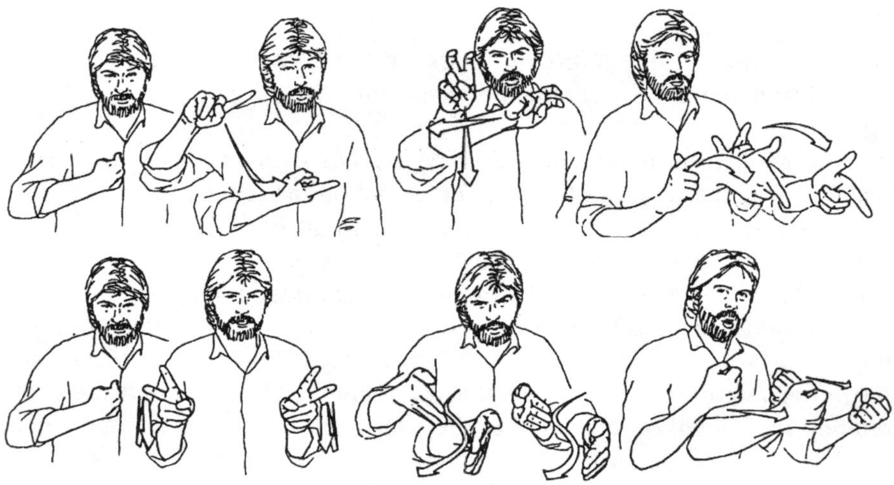

Figure 3.10 The use of facial expression in conditional clauses in DGS

____________________________Bedingungssatz
ICH NOCHMAL SCHWEIZ FAHREN-NACH, ICH DIESELBE STRECKE AUTO-FAHREN *phhh*

The German meaning of the sentence is 'Wenn ich wieder einmal in die Schweiz komme, dann nehme ich wieder dieselbe Strecke.' (= 'If I come to Switzerland again, I will take the same route.'). As can be seen in the pictures, the signer has raised eyebrows, his eyes are wide open and his head is slightly tilted while signing the conditional sentence. At the beginning of the main sentence his facial expression becomes less tense and he leans backwards. Although there are signs for the conjunction 'wenn' (= 'if') in DGS, it would be more idiomatic to use facial expression only in order to express the change from subordinate to main clause. Prillwitz states this, too:

> [...] In der deutschen Lautsprache werden Bedingungssätze meist mit dem Bindewort *wenn* eingeleitet. Eine entsprechende Bindegebärde kennt auch die DGS. Sie ist eindeutig von dem Wort *wenn* abgeleitet: Der Zeigefinger berührt die Nase an der Seite (= Kennzeichnung des Nasallautes in *wenn*). Um einen Bedingungssatz eindeutig zu kennzeichnen, verfügt die DGS jedoch auch über eigene Mittel. Wie unser Beispielsatz zeigt, wird auch hier wieder die Mimik eingesetzt. [...] (Prillwitz 1985:57)

> [...] In spoken German, conditional sentences are usually introduced by the conjunction *wenn*. A corresponding conjunctional sign is also present in DGS. It is obviously derived from the word *wenn*: the index finger touches the side of the nose (indicating the nasal in *wenn*). However, in order to unambiguously mark a conditional sentence, there are also language inherent means in DGS. Our sample sentence shows that facial expression is utilized as well. [...]

Similarly, in ASL, the manual conditional markers I-F and SUPPOSE do exist, too; but their use is optional.

Finally, it is sometimes argued that there are different non-manuals for different kinds of conditionals. Thus, Dachkovsky and Sandler (2007) observed that in IsSL, neutral or factual conditionals are marked by brow raise only, while counterfactual conditionals are marked by layered non-manuals, namely a squint and a brow raise. Their analysis of the correlations of sentence structures' pragmatic functions and non-manuals was already elaborated on above. In this context, it is obvious why in counterfactual conditional clauses (in which knowledge to the contrary of the proposition of the if-clause is entailed), have to be accompanied by a squint. The speaker appeals to some shared background knowledge which has to be present for a counterfactual conditional to work. An example from Dachkovsky and Sandler (2007:28) illustrates this.

```
      ____________brow raise+squint
(14)  IF GOALKEEPER HE CATCH-BALL, WIN GAME WIN            [IsSL]
      'If the goalkeeper had caught the ball, (the team) would have won the
      game.'
```

In this case, the addressee's knowledge of the goalkeeper not catching the ball is presupposed by the speaker. Thus the squint becomes necessary in the sentence. Dachkovsky and Sandler (2007) and Sandler (2012), e.g., also linked the different kinds of non-manuals and their correlation with certain syntactic patterns to intonational patterns which are often closely linked to syntax. This is analyzed in the subsequent section.

3.1.2.3. Facial Expression and Prosody

The last level to be mentioned at which facial expression is crucial in sign languages is the prosodic level. It is sometimes hard to distinguish whether a certain non-manual correlates with syntactic or prosodic structure in sign languages, but Sandler (2012:59) solves this apparent controversy by stating that "prosodic constituents are related to syntactic ones but are not always coextensive with them". Before discussing evidence for the link between non-manual markers and prosody, it should be mentioned that in sign languages just as in spoken languages, prosodic chunks are organized according to the prosodic hierarchy according to Selkirk (1984) (cited in Pfau and Quer (2010:397)).

syllable > foot > prosodic word > phonological phrase > intonational phrase > phonological utterance

Concerning terminology, some researchers, such as Sandler and Lillo-Martin (2006) argued that the term "intonation" is not adequate for sign languages as it is too closely linked to pitch in spoken languages. Hence, they introduced the term "superarticulation" to refer to the array of superarticulatory non-manual features that accompany manual signs in sign languages (Sandler & Lillo-Martin 2006:257). Sandler (2012) reintroduces the term intonation. Similar to terminological controversies concerning "phonology" vs. "cherology" in sign languages, I have decided to adopt the term "intonation" for this book in order to stress its comparability to spoken language intonational phenomena.

The parallels between spoken and sign language intonation are noteworthy. Thus, the illocutionary, pragmatic and semantic functions are the same, componentiality exists in both spoken and signed languages and the prosodic constituents (the phonological phrase and the intonational phrase) exist in both modalities. However, due to the anatomical predisposition of the human body, and for modality-dependent reasons, differences between the two systems are found as well. Contrasting with spoken languages that can only make use of the vocal cords, there is more than one articulator, i.e. the different movements of the articulators in sign languages (such as the brows, the lips, etc.) may potentially result in a richer intonational system.

This, however, has not been empirically researched yet (Sandler & Lillo-Martin 2006:261). One of the results of the variety of articulators in signed languages has been attested though: the simultaneous arrangement of intonational features, where simultaneity refers to two different things. Firstly, the superarticulations are arranged simultaneously to the manual features or text, and secondly, they are arranged simultaneously to each other. This kind of organization is not possible in spoken languages. An example of the layering of non-manual features (not only facial expression) in intonation can be seen below (taken with slight changes from Sandler & Lillo-Martin 2006:256).

(15)

	[[BOOK-THERE]$_P$ [INDEX$_3$ WRITE]$_P$]$_{INT}$	[[INTERESTING]$_P$]$_{INT}$
brows	______________________________up	__________down
eyes	__________squint	__________droop
mouth	____________'O'	__________down
head	______________________________tilt	
mouthing	__________'book'	___'interesting'
torso	_____________________________lean	

As is clear above, intonation in sign languages is componential. This means that non-manual arrays usually consist of more than one non-manual feature of which each one is meaning-bearing. Each feature has a more or less fixed meaning, i.e. that certain facial expressions seem to be linked to certain pragmatic functions (Sandler 2012). This was already mentioned for the correlation between facial expression and syntax as in conditionals, for example. However, the facial expressions observed in many of the above mentioned sentence types, could also be interpreted as intonational contours. Thus a brow raise and wide eyes (and a forward head position) that are usually used in yes/no questions could be equaled with a rising pitch contour (high tone) that is almost universally found in spoken languages (Bolinger 1989). Contrary to spoken languages, where the pitch contour usually only occurs on the last syllable of the prosodic phrase, non-manuals in sign languages spread over a whole sign or clause. Nevertheless, prosodic constituents are not isomorphic with syntactic constituents, i.e. the prosodic word and the morphosyntactic word do not always coincide. This is the same in spoken languages as can be seen in (16) below (example taken from Sandler & Lillo-Martin 2006:264).

(16) <u>Syntactic</u>: [This is [the cat that killed [the rat that ate [the malt]]]]
<u>Prosodic</u>: [This is the cat] [that killed the rat] [that ate the malt]

The same phenomenon can be observed in sign languages. In spoken languages, it is very common for unstressed function words to group together with a nearby prosodic word through the process of cliticization, thus forming a new prosodic word. This can be observed in sign languages, too, where personal pronouns may assimilate to a neighbouring lexical sign by change of handshape (e.g. Sandler 1999; 2012).

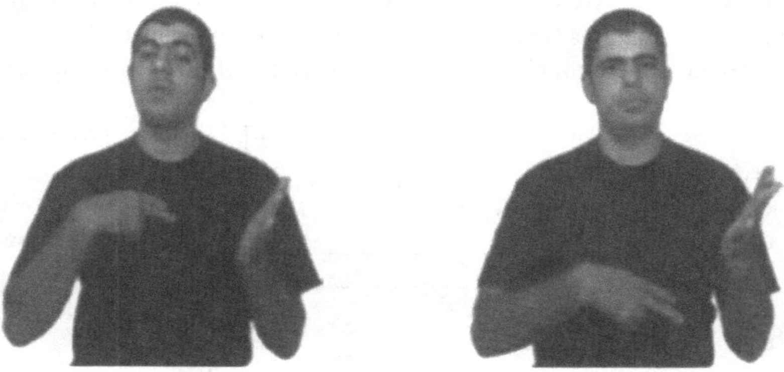

Figure 3.11 The IsSL signs I and I-READ

The above figure from Sandler and Lillo-Martin (2006:248) shows the IsSL 1SG personal pronoun and the assimilated handshape on the right in I-READ.[35]

As becomes evident from this rather brief sketch of prosody in signed languages, facial expression may relate to intonation and prosodic constituents in sign languages rather than to syntactic constituents. However, as was already mentioned above, it is often not easy to clearly distinguish prosodic and syntactic constituents. The examples mentioned in this section provide some evidence for facial expression being linked to intonation. Further research in this area is needed in order to clarify the remaining unresolved issues.

3.1.3. Head Movements

Head nods and head shakes can be used similarly by speakers of spoken and signed languages. Thus, Sutton-Spence and Woll (2006:92) mention that head nods may be used to signal 'yes' or agreement in BSL without using any manual sign at all. In many spoken languages, head nods signal agreement, too. Moreover, they mention head nods as an important feature of BSL that signals attention during a conversation, making a head nod in these situations a discourse feature. Apart from these discourse or non-grammatical functions, head nods, shakes and tilts have grammatical functions which will be discussed in turn below.

One of the functions of head nods in BSL mentioned by Sutton-Spence and Woll (2006) is the indication of the first person. In this case, the manual sign for the first person singular becomes oblivious and can be discarded with altogether. Moreover, fast head nods indicate that a signer insists on the truth of an utterance. Phenomena like this are encountered in spoken languages as well. Thus, fast head nods are similar to French *si* or Portuguese *é*. Sutton-Spence and Woll (2006:92) mention the example of fast head nods in the sentence CAT DOG CHASE which means 'Yes, the cat did definitely chase the dog, no matter what you think.'

Finally, single or successive small nods may be used to indicate that the information given in an utterance is complete or that a comment upon a certain statement is complete. Sutton-Spence and Woll (2006:93) mention the example FLY LONDON ATHENS followed by a small head nod, AEROPLANE LAND followed by a small head nod. In this case, the head nods both indicate that the piece of information given is complete. It is also argued that in ASL, predicates of a conditional clause are often accompanied by a head thrust (Pfau & Quer 2010:389).

A side-to-side headshake is closely linked to negation in sign languages. Most sign languages studied so far have a non-manual means to negate sentences (Pfau & Quer 2010). However, the distribution of these head shakes is different cross-linguistically. The most common patterns that can be observed in ASL, e.g., are a side-to-side head shake that either accompanies the manual negation particle only or spreads over the whole VP. The manual megation particle is not obligatory in this case. The non-manual feature alone suffices to negate the sentence. The option without the manual component seems to be favoured by most sign languages. The different ways to negate a sentence in ISL were already discussed in chapter 2.6. In case no negation particle is present, the non-manual has to spread over the VP (Pfau & Quer 2010:386). An example from ASL can be seen below (taken from Pfau & Quer 2010:387).

              __hs ____[__hs]
(17) a. JOHN NOT BUY HOUSE [ASL]
'John didn't buy the house.'

              _______hs
b. JOHN BUY HOUSE [ASL]
'John didn't buy the house.'

Some sign languages, however, show different patterns for the non-manual only options. In LSC, e.g., it is possible that the head shake only accompanies the predicate.

Yet another, completely different type of sign languages with respect to negation, are "manually dominant" sign languages (Zeshan 2006). In these sign languages it is ungrammatical to negate a sentence by using a head shake alone. Sign languages of that kind are for example HKSL and LIS. In other sign languages such as Turkish Sign Language (TSL), e.g., a backward head tilt is more common in order to negate a sentence and co-exists with a head shake (Pfau & Quer 2010:387).

Moreover, Sutton-Spence and Woll (2006) mention a side-to-side head shake as a means to respond in the negative to a yes/no question, as a means of negation of rhetorical questions, to negate a topic and to negate a whole clause in BSL. This could be seen in example (17b). In most of these cases, there is no form of manual negation, the head shake suffices in order to express the negative.

Beside the grammatical functions of head shakes mentioned above, head shakes can also express emotions such as regret, frustration, disbelief or sorrow (Sutton-Spence & Woll 2006:94). An example of this (taken from Sutton-Spence & Woll 2006:94) can be seen in (18) below.

hs (over GONE)

(18) GROUP LEAVE NINE-O'CLOCK ARRIVE ME FIVE-PAST NINE GONE [BSL]
'The group left at nine o'clock, and I arrived at five past nine, to find them gone.'

Finally, it seems noteworthy that topics are often marked by head tilts or specific head positions in many sign languages of the world such as ASL or HKSL. However, head tilts usually do not serve as the only topic marker but are layered with other non-manual components such as brow raises, for instance. As this was already outlined in detail in section 3.1.2.2, I will not elaborate on this again.

3.2. Mouth Actions

Almost forty years after the beginning of extensive research on mouth actions especially in European sign languages, mouth patterns are still a controversial topic among sign linguists. As yet, researchers have been unable to define the exact nature and functions of the different kinds of mouth actions.

Especially in ASL, mouth actions are an under-researched topic because mouthings in particular have been rejected by many. A study by Nadolske and Rosenstock (2007) has acknowledged the existence and importance of mouthings in ASL and demanded further investigations into that direction. Differences in frequency and usage seem to be due to a high or low degree of cross-modal language contact, especially with respect to oralist education policies in deaf schools.

Despite these controversies, a general consensus on the classification of mouth actions into at least two different categories has been reached (e.g. Boyes Braem & Sutton-Spence 2001; Crasborn et al. 2008; Bank et al. 2011; Mohr 2012). There are "spoken components" which are said to be derived from the surrounding spoken language, and "oral components", formed within a sign language and thus sign language inherent (Sutton-Spence & Woll 2006; Crasborn et al. 2008; Bank et al. 2011). The terms "mouthings" for spoken components and "mouth gestures" for oral components are nowadays widely used (e.g. Raino 2001; Sutton-Spence & Day 2001; Crasborn et al. 2008; Bank et al. 2011; Mohr 2012). I have adopted the latter terminology for my book and will refer to spoken components as "mouthings" and to oral components as "mouth gestures". Schermer (1990) identified at least three different functions of mouth actions in sign languages. They are **disambiguation** (of homonyms like BRUDER/SCHWESTER ('brother/sister') in DGS), **meaning specification** and **sole carrier of meaning** (as adverbs, for instance).

In the following sections, I will elaborate on the different kinds of mouth actions referring to the established dichotomy. I will discuss mouth gestures first and subsequently elaborate on a special kind of mouth gesture called "echo phonology". In chapter 3.2.3 I will concentrate on mouthings. Finally, in 3.2.4, the form and functions of spread mouthings are treated.

3.2.1. Mouth Gestures

As already mentioned in the previous section, mouth gestures are inherent in sign language, they have always belonged to the linguistic system of sign languages. Mouth gestures do not seem to be derived from or related to spoken language words. In general, a mouth gesture can be defined as a mouth pattern that either changes or remains constant during the articulation of a sign (Pfau & Quer 2010). Thus, in the DGS sign HABEN ('have'), the hand (>-hand) performs no movement except for a wriggling of the fingers, the mouth gesture is "shhhhhhhhh" (constant mouth gesture). In the

BSL sign DISAPPEAR, the manual components (a closing of the hands and an abrupt final stop) are echoed by the mouth gesture starting as an interdental fricative and ending in a bilabial stop (Crasborn et al. 2008:49) (changing mouth gesture). The latter kind of mouth gesture will be treated in detail in section 3.2.2 on echo phonology.

While a more general distinction between mouthings and mouth gestures is made by almost all researchers in the field (e.g. Raino 2001; Boyes Braem 2001; Lewin & Schembri 2011), Crasborn and colleagues (2008) introduced a more fine-grained distinction of four different kinds of mouth gestures. They distinguish between "adverbial mouth gestures", "semantically empty mouth gestures", "enacting mouth gestures" and "mouth activity in the context of whole face activity" (Crasborn et al. 2008:49ff) according to the lexical and morphosyntactic properties of these groups. The different categories of mouth gestures will be defined in turn in the following.

Adverbial mouth gestures specify adverbial information additional to that specified by a manual sign (Crasborn et al. 2008:49). This category was also identified by Sutton-Spence and Woll (2006:86f) as "manner and degree adverbs". It seems to be present in most sign languages, and has been identified in many sign languages known to date including ASL, BSL and Swedish Sign Language (SSL).

From a morphological point of view, these adverbs could be analyzed as bound morphemes because they usually combine with the manual component of the sign. They add information on the manner or effort of an action as well as indicating the size of an object or the degree of an adjective. Thus, the mouth gestures might not exclusively be used in order to modify a verbal sign but also in order to modify a nominal sign and thus fulfill adjectival instead of adverbial function. Some researchers include adjectival mouth actions in this category if they are productive (Sutton-Spence & Woll 2006:86). A typical example of a manner and degree adverbial mouth gesture are puffed cheeks meaning 'large, long' in DGS.

Semantically empty mouth gestures may be obligatory in signs in order to guarantee well-formedness but do not carry extra or independent meaning (Schermer 1990, Crasborn et al. 2008:49). Usually, the movement of the mouth parallels the movement of the hands and never opposes it. The above mentioned BSL sign DISAPPEAR is an example of this kind of mouth gesture. These signs have been analyzed as echo phonology by Woll (2001) and will be elaborated on in section 3.2.2.

In **enacting mouth gestures** the mouth performs real actions such as laughing, vomiting, biting (although sometimes in a stylized way) and can thus function as the sole articulator. These mouth gestures may accompany a manual sign as for instance a chewing movement that accompanies the sign CHEWING, or they may be the sole articulator of an action as in LAUGH (Crasborn et al. 2008). The latter kind seems more complex, as it is not frequently attested in earlier stages of sign language development as in younger sign languages such as Mauritian Sign Language (MSL) (Adone et al. 2009).

Mouth actions as part of overall facial expression shall only be elaborated on very briefly here. They will not be relevant for the analysis of the collected data for the reasons mentioned in the following.

Certain mouth actions appear as part of, as Crasborn and colleagues call it, "a global facial expression" (Crasborn et al. 2008:50). In this case, the mouth is active during sign production but is not independent of facial expression as in other cases. This kind of action has to be considered as one special kind of mouth gesture (Crasborn et al. 2008). Mouth actions in the context of overall facial expression often occur with an affective rather than a grammatical meaning as in the example of the expression of disgust where the mouth is involved but has no independent role (Crasborn et al. 2008:51). They might also be part of the phonology of the sign as in signs like SAD. Because of the often non-grammatical meaning of the mouth actions, they have been left out of the current investigation.

A final issue that seems noteworthy in regard to mouth gestures is the fact that their frequency seems related to the morphological complexity of a sign. Thus, they occur more frequently with morphologically complex signs (Adone et al. 2009) such as verbs and especially classifiers for example. This has been found for other sign languages like SSL, NGT and BSL as well (Crasborn et al. 2008). However, verbs have proven to be a somewhat difficult matter. Bank et al. (2011) report that high frequency NGT verbs can be combined with either a mouth gesture or a Dutch mouthing. Moreover, while verbs have been divided into different types as for example in the Nadolske and Rosenstock study (2007) (they categorized verbs into directional verbs, aspect verbs, plain verbs and modal verbs) other studies such as Crasborn et al. (2008) and Adone et al. (2009) did not subdivide the verb classes. Certainly, the differences concerning the matter of classification of verbs depend on the focus of each single study. An in-depth study of the distribution of mouth actions with respect to different verb types remains to be done. However, inter- as well as intra-linguistic variation is to be expected. A preliminary analysis for ISL is discussed in 6.2.3.

After the description of the different kinds of mouth gestures, a special analysis of one kind of mouth gesture, namely enacting mouth gestures, will be described in more detail under the heading "echo phonology" (Woll 2001).

3.2.2. Echo Phonology

The theory of echo phonology was first elaborated in Woll's 2001 article "The Sign That Dares to Speak Its Name: Echo Phonology in British Sign Language (BSL)" (Boyes Braem & Sutton-Spence (2001), pp. 87–98). It refers to a special kind of mouth gesture that has so far only been researched for BSL. Woll's theory will be outlined in the following.

Her account is based on the fact that there are different kinds of mouth gestures, namely constant and changing mouth gestures, as already outlined in section 3.2.1. While in constant mouth gestures the position of the mouth is held constant throughout the articulation of the manual sign, in changing mouth gestures the mouth configuration usually changes during the articulation of the manual. Woll (2001:90) observes that constant mouth gestures usually occur with adverbials (such as "tense spread lips" in BSL). In contrast, echo phonology mouth gestures usually occur with a changing mouth gesture (Woll 2001:91). Another defining feature of echo phonology mouth gestures, according to Woll, is that they occur in the citation form of signs and that they are obligatory for the sign to be well-formed, i.e. they are part of the phonology of the sign. The characteristic of these mouth actions that led Woll to call them echo phonology, is that these kinds of mouth gestures always mirror or echo the manual movements of the manual sign (Woll 2001:91). This is in line with the well-known fact that manual and oral actions are often well coordinated (Nobe 1996). However, contrasting with spoken languages where the mouth is the driving force for accompanying gestures of the hands, in echo phonology the hands "drive" the mouth. The example of the BSL sign SUCCEED shows that the thumbs are initially in contact and move apart abruptly while the mouth articulates /pa/. (Woll 2001:92) contrasts this with an impossible version of SUCCEED in BSL because the signer inhales which opposes the movement of the hands.

Woll identified a number of recurring elements for echo phonology in BSL. In order to provide an overview of the elements that have been attested, some of them are mentioned below. It is noteworthy that almost all listed items involve articulations at the front of the mouth or lips because they are most visible at that point (Woll 2001:92, f.). Some of the consonants (in syllable initial and final position) that have been observed are /p/ and /m/ and the vocalics /y/, /w/ and /u/. Woll also mentions exhalation and inhalation breath patterns (Woll 2001:93).

The theory elaborated above may provide further insights into research areas such as the structure of the sign syllable, sonority and language evolution. Echo phonology provides the opportunity to gain a deeper insight into the relationship between signed and spoken language phonology because mouth movements in echo phonology are derived from the manual sign. Thus, the syllable structure of the manual component and the syllable structure of the echo component can be investigated at the same time (Woll 2001:95). Furthermore, echo theory might also contribute to the description of manual syllable structure and the sequential nature of sign syllables and sonority hierarchies in particular. Finally, Woll's theory provides a concrete example of how arbitrary spoken forms and non-arbitrary (iconic) gestural forms are interrelated.

The above discussion of echo phonology in BSL provides interesting implications for signed and spoken language research alike. A next desirable step would be an investigation of mouth gestures in other sign languages with a particular focus on echo phonology.

3.2.3. Mouthings

In spite of a large body of literature on mouth actions, the exact status, function and origins of mouthings have not been clearly determined yet. There are many different opinions concerning this phenomenon in sign languages and theories vary considerably. Bank et al. (2011: 251) describe current accounts of mouthings as a continuum ranging from mouthings as outcomes of online code-blending on the one end to mouthings as fully lexicalized items in the lexicon of a sign language on the other end. Three theories of mouthings in sign languages will be presented and placed on this continuum. Differences and similarities of current theories will be outlined subsequently.

Situated towards the end of mouthings as an outcome of online code-blending is the theory by Hohenberger and Happ (2001). The research team including Leuninger, view the phenomenon from a generativist point of view. In their 2001 paper they especially take psycholinguistic theories on language production and sociolinguistic theories of language contact into account. Their point of departure was that sign languages as minority languages have always developed in contact with the surrounding spoken languages. Thus sociolinguistic factors are highly influential as parameters such as language prestige, the distribution of linguistic and societal power, educational and teaching infrastructure and general acceptance of a signed language in society may play an important role for the use of mouthings. They also claim that the origin of mouthings is oralist education (Hohenberger & Happ 2001:155).

Hohenberger and Happ (2001:157) believe that mouthings result from mixing the spoken and signed language mode. From the standpoint of Generative Grammar, they argue that signing relates to both signed language competence and performance, mouthings however are a mere performance phenomenon (Hohenberger & Happ 2001). A fact that, according to them, substantiates their claim is that sign language can dispense with mouthings altogether which can be seen in the varying degrees of mouthings observed in different signers. These range from full to reduced to no mouthings at all. The origins of this highly varying use of mouthings in their study could not be related fully to the family situation or type of language acquisition (i.e. if the parents are hearing or deaf) as attempted. As it has generally been stated in the literature that mouthings are context dependent (e.g. Sutton-Spence & Day 2001; Nadolske & Rosenstock 2007), this could be an explanation for the varying use of mouthings as well.

Concerning the nature and frequency of mouthings, Happ and Hohenberger's findings are in line with observations from other languages such as MSL. Thus, mouthings occur mostly with nouns or lexical categories in general. Mouthings cannot occur with morphologically more complex signs because inflections seem to represent a problem for mouthings. Inflectional information is only conveyed by a sign and not by its mouthing. The most common kind of relation between mouthing and manual sign is that of semantic redundancy. This is the case when mouthing and manual sign convey the same meaning.[36] As will be shown in 6.2, this view seems rather controversial and far from actual linguistic reality.

Summarizing, in Hohenberger & Happ's account, mouthings are viewed not as an integral part of sign languages, but merely as a peripheral performance phenomenon. They can be dispensed with and only came into sign languages via language contact. In light of the findings from ISL that are presented in chapters 4, 5 and 6, these claims are highly doubtful.

A somewhat intermediate account on the continuum of mouthing theories is put forward by Keller (1999; 2001). Acknowledging and searching for an explanation of the relations between mouthings and signs that vary individually, systematically and with respect to particular items, he supported a kinematic theory of mouthings. While assuming that language contact is the driving force behind mouthings in DGS, he denies that the interplay of language processing and bilingual or diglossic knowledge of German and DGS fully accounts for the data (Keller 2001:192). Relying on language acquisition data, he doubts that mouthings actually denote, as children would be unable to communicate as long as they have not mastered an assumed mouthings system. Rejecting Hohenberger and Happ's theory, he claims that their analysis is neither applicable to all sign languages, nor does it account for the nature of mouthings (Keller 2001:198, f.).

Keller mentions a whole list of problems that have seriously hampered empirical research on mouthings in sign languages. One of these problems is the great variation in the use of mouthings. This variation may be due to educational factors (such as an education under oralism or not), social factors, differences in first and second language acquisition, sign language proficiency (the frequent use of mouthings might be tied to low sign language proficiency, for example) or regional variation.

Moreover, there are several methodological problems as, for example, phonologically biased researchers and transcription problems stemming from overenthusiastic researchers who transcribe whole words of the surrounding spoken language although these are not present (Keller 2001:203, f.). This last problem is explained by the McGurk-Effect from psycholinguistics which shows that visual information often facilitates auditory perception (cf. e.g. McGurk & MacDonald 1976). This kind of perception is, however, only available to hearing people. In deaf people, he suggests, "only the visible information channel contributes to identifying a specific mouthing" (Keller 2001:205). Thus, he reasons, there is no distinction between mouthings and mouth gestures as they are both language related oral gestures. He finally states that both have to serve similar functions. However, only mouth gestures are fully lexicalized while mouthings are purely kinematic in nature. He puts forward the hypothesis that mouthings will drop out of a sign language in the course of its development. This view does not apply to ISL, as will be shown in chapter 5.3.

Furthermore, he elaborates in his empirical research on possible combinations of mouthings and signs. These are: sign + no mouthing, sign + mouthing, sign + several mouthings, no sign + mouthing and several signs + (one) mouthing, which is similar to findings in other sign languages such as NGT (Crasborn et al. 2008; Bank et al. 2011). He cites findings from acquisition research showing that mouthings are acquired holistically and are not segmental, which would actually classify them as gestures instead of linguistic material.

In conclusion, Keller proposes an innovative investigation method for the phenomenon of mouthings. The most important point of his account is the supposed kinematic as opposed to segmental nature of mouthings. This view is certainly interesting as it resolves some of the unresolved issues in other theories of mouthings. However, further research, especially in the field of sign language acquisition, is needed in order to substantiate his claim.

Ebbinghaus and Heßmann (e.g. 1994; 1996; 2001) conducted extensive research on mouthings in DGS. They view sign language as a form of multi-dimensional communication, of which mouthings constitute one part. They do not believe that manual signs are the words of sign languages, a view that is common among sign linguists (Ebbinghaus & Heßmann 2001:133). They state that manual signs and non-manuals are separate parts of a single unit, especially emphasizing that non-manual signs are meaningful, which is in line with the different linguistic and discourse functions of non-manuals discussed in chapter 3.1. What seems important in this context is the claim that mouthings are different from non-manuals proper (Ebbinghaus & Heßmann 2001:133). While other researchers have adopted this view and it seems to be reasonable at least for DGS, it is doubtful whether this actually applies to ISL as well (cf. chapter 4). In ISL it seems that although etymologically different, mouthings are non-manual features just like mouth gestures, eye gaze, etc.

Furthermore, Ebbinghaus and Heßmann (2001:134) suggest adding information on obligatory non-manual signs to the lexicographic information about a manual sign. According to them, DGS is a language that exists across different modalities and signers use mouthings as an additional source of information for an otherwise semantically under-determined manual sign (Ebbinghaus & Heßmann 2001). The semantic function of mouthings is readily acknowledged while syntactic or grammatical functions of mouthings are challenged. Thus, the disambiguating function of mouthings in homonyms is supported whereas grammatical functions of mouthings are not mentioned. The controversial nature of this claim will be shown in chapter 4, as especially the phenomenon of spread mouth actions reveals crucial syntactic functions of mouthings (as well as mouth gestures).

Concerning the origins and functions of mouthings, Ebbinghaus and Heßmann do not believe that mouthings can be regarded as instances of code-mixing or borrowing as many other researchers do. That would only be the case if the mouthings were spoken language words intruding in the sign language context. They believe that mouthings belong to the sign language context (Ebbinghaus & Heßmann 2001); the context is just unique for the use of spoken words. The mouthed words are often not German (or taken from the ambient spoken language) proper (Ebbinghaus & Heßmann 1996). They are only similar to or fragments of a spoken language word and can only be recognized as a certain spoken language word because they are contextualized by the manual sign.

As is evident above, Ebbinghaus and Heßmann clearly view mouthings as a part of sign languages. According to them, they are just one of many components that add to the multidimensional communication mode of a sign language.

Despite the controversy on the origins and functions of mouthings, there are certain facts that are universally agreed on. Most researchers today concur that mouthings originated as borrowings from spoken languages (e.g. Raino 2001; Boyes Braem 2001; Sutton-Spence & Woll 2006; Nadolske & Rosenstock 2007). The functionality of mouthings varies across different sign languages. Thus, the function of disambiguation of homonyms as in the aforementioned DGS example of BRUDER/SCHWESTER is uncontroversial for DGS, a sign language that has had a lot of contact with the surrounding spoken language due to an oralist education policy in the last decades. In cases like these, mouthings seem to substitute lexical variation in manual signs. However, it is possible that with an expanding lexicon these mouthings would become unnecessary and fall out of use. In contrast to the situation described for DGS and several other European sign languages, mouthings have been described as very restricted in ASL (e.g. Padden 1980; Boyes Braem 2001). Consequently, their functions remain controversial.

For the lexical level, Boyes Braem (2001) also reports that mouthings may function as gap filling mechanisms in DSGS. This might refer to the linguistic system in general, or to an individual's language use, especially with respect to later learners.

Furthermore, mouthings might fulfill the function of grammatical derivation. Hence, they act as derivational elements used for the creation of new lexical material (Boyes Braem 2001). These items are usually nominal in character (Schermer 1990; Boyes Braem 2001; Nadolske & Rosenstock 2007; Crasborn et al. 2008; Bank et al. 2011) which is supported by theories on spoken language mixing (Poplack & Meechan 1998). Another phenomenon that has been observed for several sign languages is the link of mouthings to the morphological complexity of a sign or open and closed class differences. Thus, morphologically simple signs (usually nouns and adjectives) occur more often with mouthings while morphologically complex signs occur more often with mouth gestures (Crasborn et al. 2008; Sutton-Spence & Day 2001). Crasborn et al. (2008) state that mouthings are most frequent with nouns and uninflected verbs, open class items and morphologically simple signs, which is supported by their findings for NGT, BSL and SSL where mouthings occur most often with content items (nouns, verbs, adverbs and adjectives) (Crasborn et al. 2008:53). All three languages investigated by them show similar figures for the word class of nouns, for instance: BSL 40%, NGT 39%, SSL 43%. As will be shown in 3.2.4, mouthings may also function to bind syntactic elements from different word classes by the process of spreading.

Finally, mouthings have been thought to fulfil certain discourse functions such as "constructed speaking" which refers to the imitation of spoken language as used by hearing people and drawing attention to a certain part of a narrative (Boyes Braem 2001).

In spite of the similarities mentioned above, there is a lot of inter- as well as intra-linguistic variation which makes it hard to determine the exact function and status of mouthings. As was already shown in the description of Keller's theory, there is more than one possible combination of manual sign and mouthing. Even mouthings which do not accompany any manual sign are possible. Vogt-Svendsen (2001) even mentions what she calls "simultaneous compound signs". In this case, the mouthings function as non-manual adjectives modifying the nominal manual sign. Thus, in Norwegian Sign Language (NSL) the sign PULLOVER might be accompanied by the mouthing *rød* (='red') expressing the meaning 'red pullover'. These types of compounds are similar to grammatical derivation by mouthings, as new lexical material is created.

Moreover, Sutton-Spence and Day (2001) and Nadolske and Rosenstock (2007) found striking differences concerning the use of mouthings in different registers and/or text types. For BSL, e.g., 77% mouthings were found for informative registers and only 50% mouthings for narrative registers (Sutton-Spence & Day 2001). Nadolske and Rosenstock investigated mouthing behaviour in ASL for lectures, natural conversation and story-telling. They found that the categories of lecture and natural conversation were fairly similar concerning the use of mouthings (average of 60.4%), however, the occurrence of mouthings in story-telling was much lower (42.4%). This refutes their own and other researchers' theories that the frequency of mouthings increases with the formality of the situation. Yet, investigations into that direction have to prove this fact for other sign languages.

The form of mouthings may also differ inter- as well as intra-linguistically. Thus, mouthings may be either reduced or full. A whole spoken language word that is mouthed alongside a manual sign such as for example *Bruder* being mouthed to accompany the manual sign BRUDER ('brother') in DGS is referred to as a full mouthing. A reduced mouthing refers to a spoken language word of which only a part (often the first syllable) is articulated alongside the manual sign as in the example *zoek-* (from the Dutch word *zoeken* = 'to look for') that accompanies the NGT sign ZOEKEN (Crasborn et al. 2008). Bank et al. (2011) further report that in NGT, the stressed syllables of Dutch words are usually retained in mouthings, while unstressed syllables might get lost.

Recent studies (e.g. Crasborn et al. 2008) have also investigated the spreading of mouthings. This is the last issue in this section and will be dealt with in section 3.2.4, together with the spreading of mouth gestures.

3.2.4. Spreading of Mouth Actions

Although spreading of mouth actions has been mentioned in the literature on mouth action research, the first detailed study on the spreading behavior of the different types of mouth actions was the Crasborn et al. study from 2008. It was also the first larger cross-linguistic study on this phenomenon, although other studies had certainly mentioned it and provided examples from different sign languages (e.g. Plaza Pust 2005; Pfau 2005; 2009). Other studies such as Sandler (1999) had looked at spreading of mouthings for one sign language (IsSL in this case) only. Crasborn and colleagues investigated whether all types of mouth actions spread, whether the direction of spreading is the same cross-linguistically, and they investigated the spreading domain in further detail looking at its size (Crasborn et al. 2008:56). With their results they hoped to gain further insight into signed languages' prosodic phonology. I will mainly concentrate on this study, as it is most informative concerning the spread of mouth actions across language boundaries.

Before elaborating on a discussion of spreading of mouth actions in sign languages, I will address some parallels to spreading of tone in spoken languages. Pfau (2009) mentions these parallels of "tone sandhi" in spoken languages and the spreading of non-manual features in sign languages. Concerning spoken languages, there are three possible ways in which tones may spread. Firstly, a tone may spread onto a toneless segment as in Chilungu (a Bantu language of the Niger-Congo phylum), where the high (register) tone of the prefix *kú-* may spread to all adjacent syllables (except for the last one) as in *kú-vúl-à=* 'to be enough' or *kú-sóóbólól-à=* 'to sort out' (Bickmore 1996: 11).

Secondly, a tone may spread and combine with the tone of the adjacent unit, thus creating a contour tone. In Yoruba (a Benue-Congo language of the Niger-Congo phylum), high and low level tones never combine in bisyllabic words. The tone of the first syllable spreads onto the second syllable resulting in a contour tone (Pfau 2009). This can be seen in /àlá/, [àlâ] = 'dream' or /rárà/, [rárâ] = 'elegy' (Yip 2002: 47).

Finally, spreading of tone might also involve delinking, resulting in a tone-bearing unit losing its tone (Pfau 2009). Hence, in Barasana (a language of the southern branch of the Tucanoan language family) compounds, the last tone of the first part of the compound spreads onto the second part. An example of this is *héè + jáí–>héèjàì=* 'shaman (ancestor-jaguar)' (Gomez-Imbert & Kenstowicz 2000: 433).

As could be seen in the above examples, tone easily spreads word-internally. The same holds true for word-external spreading onto clitics, for instance. This kind of spreading is similar to the spread of non-manuals in sign languages, as discussed for mouth actions in the following paragraphs.[37]

Crasborn et al. (2008) as well as Pfau (2009) found that mouth actions in sign languages may spread onto adjacent functional signs such as pronouns, for example. Especially mouthings (as they often co-occur with nouns or other content words), often spread onto functional signs. Crasborn et al. (2008) found that mouthings spread in a manner similar to mouth gestures (being sign language inherent), a fact which, according to them, proves that mouthings fulfill a grammatical function in sign languages and are not due to code-switching (Crasborn et al. 2008:57). However, spread mouth gestures were rare in all three sign languages (SSL, BSL, NGT) investigated. Moreover, intra-linguistic variation was observed concerning this issue as some signers did not use spread mouth gestures at all.

The direction of spreading was very different for the sign languages investigated. BSL showed a pattern of rightward (progressive) spreading, NGT an overall rightward pattern while the data for SSL was very mixed. One of the signers showed as much leftward as rightward spreading while the other signer showed much less leftward spreading. They analyzed the data with respect to two hypotheses. The first is that spreading proceeds from content to function words which is supported by the finding that almost all spreading, irrespective of the direction, went from content words (such as nouns) to function words (such as determiners). The second hypothesis is that mouth actions may spread according to prosodic binding (Boyes Braem 2001) similar to prosodic binding in spoken (tone) languages.[38] This theory suggests the prosodic linking of signs to form a syntactic unit (Crasborn et al. 2008:64).

The results were very heterogeneous as in BSL, spreading appears to be strictly rightward, irrespective of the type of sign (content or function). The SSL data could not be accounted for by a content-to-function word hypothesis as for example compound signs (morphological units) that were linked by mouth actions could not be explained. Thus the prosodic binding theory seems to be more likely for SSL. In NGT, mouth actions seem to conform to the content-to-function word hypothesis. This might cause leftward (regressive) spreading which is not avoided as in BSL, however it is much rarer than rightward spreading (Crasborn et al. 2008:65).

As spreading was observed not only onto the adjacent sign but over more than one neighbouring sign, a claim for the existence of not only prosodic words but also prosodic phrases was made. However, further research in this area is needed to prove or disprove these preliminary findings. Similarly, research on the spreading behaviour of mouth actions in other sign languages is needed in order to investigate whether the direction of spreading is a sign language specific feature or not. The issue of spreading of mouth actions is also discussed regarding the ISL data in chapter 4.2.1. It will be shown that especially theories of prosodic binding seem to be well-substantiated claims.

Chapter 4
Mouth Actions in ISL – A Typology of Mouthings and Mouth Gestures

While mouth actions have been researched for many European sign languages and some studies on mouth actions in non-European sign languages, such as MSL, exist (Adone et al. 2009), the topic of mouth actions in ISL has not been researched empirically so far. However, mouth actions are frequently acknowledged in the literature on ISL, as e.g. in Ó Baoill and Matthews (2000). These studies mostly mention mouth gestures though, while the topic of mouthings is often rather marginal: "Today a certain amount of lip-patterns may be observed co-occurring with manual productions" (Ó Baoill & Matthews 2000:11). In this citation, Ó Baoill and Matthews refer to English language words being mouthed (mouthings) while performing the manual sign when using the term "lip-patterns". However, in other works the term "lip patterns" may refer to mouth gestures instead. As can be seen, terminology for the different kinds of mouth actions often varies and is not consistent in the sign linguistic literature. This work, however, tries to be consistent in using the terms mouthings and mouth gestures for the two distinct kinds of mouth actions observed introduced in 3.2.

Mouth gestures, by contrast, have been described in some more detail in several publications (e.g. Ó Baoill & Matthews 2000; Leeson & Grehan 2004). Ó Baoill and Matthews (2000:162) mention four distinct mouth patterns as "manner markers" in ISL. These are the intense marker "ee", the clumsy marker "th", the thin or delicate marker "oo" and the disappearing marker "um". Examples of all four markers can be seen in figure 4.1 (from Ó Baoill & Matthews 2000:162).

They function as adverbials, as they usually accompany a verb in order to express in which way a certain action is carried out. They might, however, also have adjectival function when describing an object, for example. The "oo" marker may be used when describing a very thin or delicate object like a thin stripe on some kind of surface such as a bowl, for instance.

Other texts mention certain mouth actions as part of parallel mouth/hand signs (Leeson & Grehan 2004:44). These signs are highly specific to a certain sign language and as idiomatic expressions, which are often very difficult to translate into a spoken or another signed language. Often their meaning can only be paraphrased in other languages. The signs Leeson and

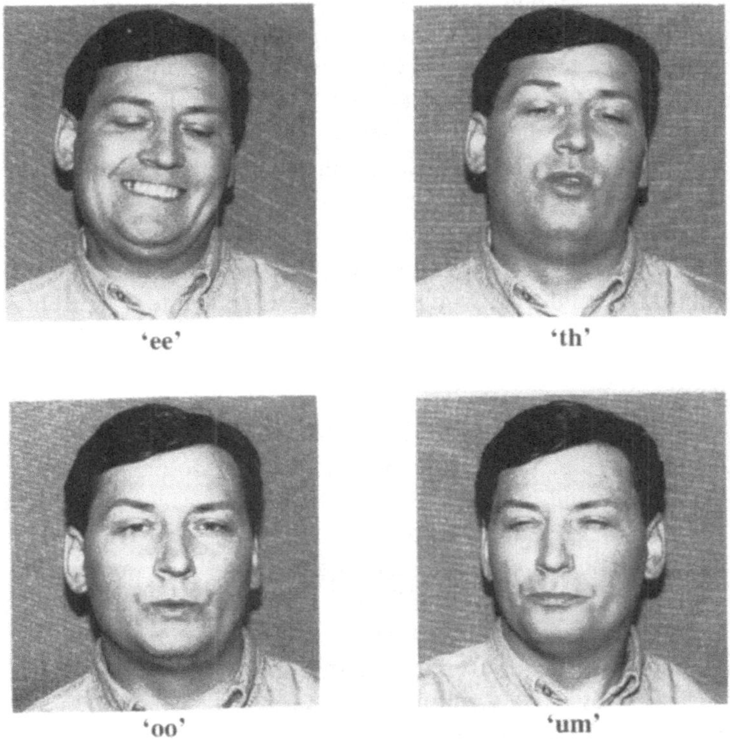

Figure 4.1 Manner markers in ISL

Grehan mention for ISL are: DON'T-LIKE$_1$ and DON'T-LIKE$_2$, SHH, FOO, DID-ON-PURPOSE, DOESN'T-SUIT-YOU/FUNNY-ON, EYEBROW-RAISE, WOF, DON'T-ANNOY-ME, UP-TO-CHIN and SPOIL. These special signs are female signs that are nowadays mostly used by elderly female signers. They occur either with special oral components that are clearly sign language inherent or one of the aforementioned manner markers. One example of this kind of co-occurrence is DON'T-LIKE$_2$ which is typically accompanied by the abovementioned intense marker "ee". The sign expresses a strong dislike of a person or a specific artistic genre (Leeson & Grehan 2004:46). It is thus logical to use the intense marker as this sign's oral component as it emphasizes the speaker's dislike of the topic of conversation. An example of a sign that is accompanied by none of the aforementioned manner markers but rather by its own "idiosyncratic" oral component is SHH. This sign is used in situations where interlocutors are at cross-purposes (Leeson & Grehan 2004:46), for example when the speaker asks the addressee to pass him the salt and the addressee hands him the pepper instead. SHH is combined with the oral component "shh".[39]

The current chapter will describe the two different kinds of mouth actions, focusing on their frequency and functions as observed in the Signs of Ireland Corpus (SOI). To this end, the chapter is subdivided into two subchapters. The first subchapter provides a description of my data sources, i.e. an outline of the corpus and methodology used in this study. The second subchapter analyzes the data in the framework of earlier mouth actions research and establishes a typology of mouthings and mouth gestures that will be used for the sociolinguistic and linguistic investigations in chapters 5 and 6.

4.1. Data Sources and Methodology

This section describes the data sources and methodology used in order to sociolinguistically and linguistically investigate the system and functions of mouth actions in ISL. The data of this study are taken from the Signs of Ireland Corpus which was kindly made available to me by the Centre for Deaf Studies at Trinity College Dublin. Data from the SOI are used with permission of the Centre for Deaf Studies, Trinity College Dublin. Special thanks to all the signers whose data I used for my study: Caroline W., Eilish B., Fergus D., Fergus M., Kevin L., Laurence H., Marian H., Michelle M., Noeleen D., Peter M., Sarah-Jane M. and Sean H. The SOI is a corpus containing self-selected personal stories, narrations of the "Frog Story" which is a story about a little boy who searches for a frog that escaped from a jar, and elicited data (the Volterra picture task was used to elicit transitive sentences).[40] Both the Frog Story and the Volterra picture task are often used in sign linguistics for data collection. The corpus comprises 40 (16=male, 24=female) ISL signers aged 18–65+. However, only very few signers are elderly (i.e. age 60+) which is going to be relevant for a differentiation into age groups later on. The data of the corpus were collected by a deaf researcher in 2004 across the Republic of Ireland. Signers are from five different locations: Dublin, Waterford, Wexford, Cork and Galway. A map of Ireland (taken from Leeson 2008) showing the locations where the data were collected is depicted in figure 4.2.

Moreover, "naive" signers were chosen for the corpus, i.e. ISL teachers or other individuals with a linguistic background were not included. All signers use ISL as their preferred language and acquired it in their youth (cf. Table 4.1).

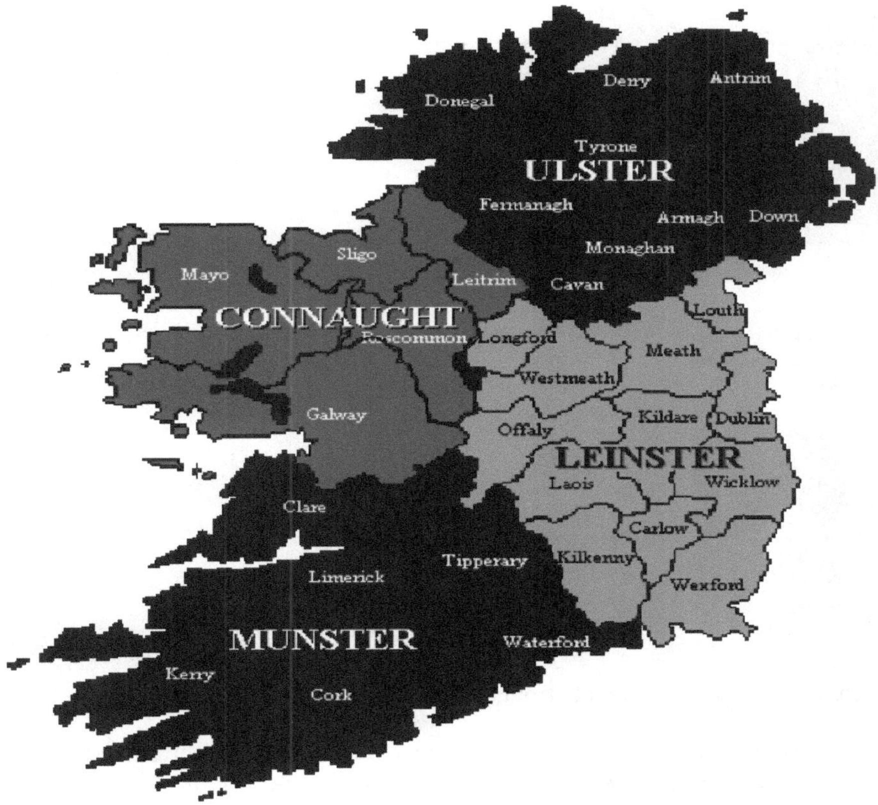

Figure 4.2 Map of Ireland

The data are digitalized and almost all 40 personal stories and 10 frog stories are annotated in ELAN. This was accomplished in 2004–2007 by three deaf researchers. ELAN (EUDICO Linguistic Annotator) was developed by the Max Planck Institute Nijmegen and is the standard tool for transcribing sign language data. For the transcription, the annotation conventions of the ECHO (European Cultural Heritage Online, http://www.let.ru.nl/signlang/echo/) Project were used. The transcriptions for the SOI generally consist of different tiers for glosses, the different non-manual features such as eye gaze or mouth actions, notes, translations and iconic information. Other special tiers have been added by different researchers working with the corpus (e.g. narrator/role shift). An example of a typical ELAN file from the SOI can be seen in figure 4.3.

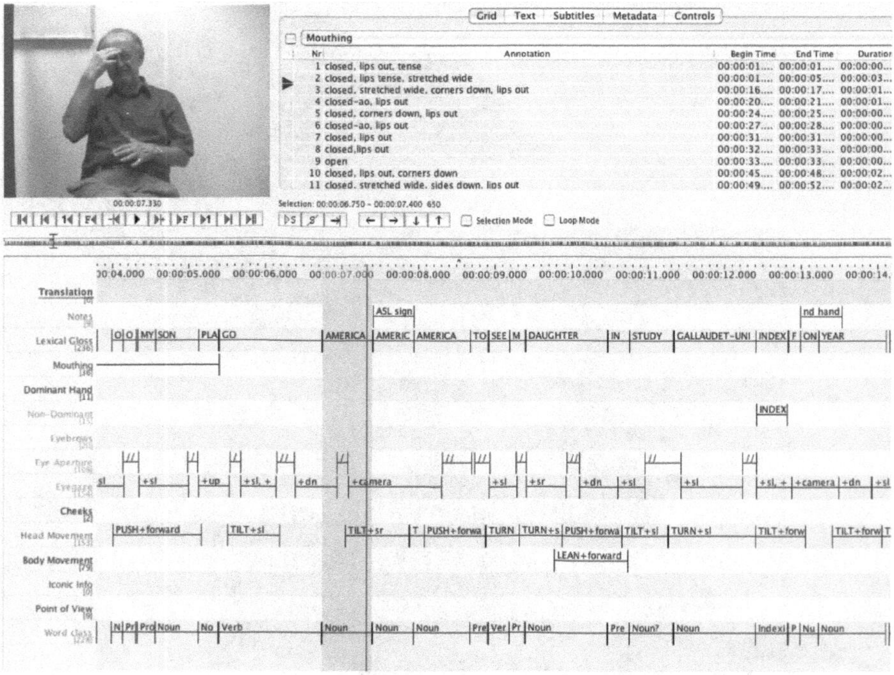

Figure 4.3 Typical ELAN file from the SOI

The data that were used for the current study on mouth actions comprised personal stories of 12 (6=male, 6=female) signers from Dublin, i.e. approximately 27 minutes of data or 2,353 signs. In order to analyze generational variation, the signers were divided into three age groups: 18–35 (age group 1), 36–50 (age group 2) and 50+ (age group 3). Each group comprises a period of 15 years, starting with age 18 which is the minimum age of the recorded signers. 15 years is a little less than 20 or 25 years that are assumed for a generation by sociological theories (e.g. Strauss & Howe 1992) or in most demographic cohorts. However, the period of 15 years seemed more adequate for this study, especially with respect to the data available in the SOI. The age range comprised in the corpus makes a distinction into 20-year intervals impossible. Moreover, there are only very few elderly signers (65+). In order to make the age groups comparable in numbers, I thus had to divide 15-year age groups. With respect to the issue of mouthing, a further age group, aged 70+ would have been ideal as male signers in this age group would have received no oral education at all and female signers would have received their primary education before the introduction of oralism at St. Mary's.[41] Unfortunately, this was not possible with the current data. Nevertheless, the majority of signers in the third age group (50+) are aged 55+. Also, many of the men in the third age group received some of their school education before the introduction of oralism at St. Joseph's, which makes a comparison of genders in this age group particularly interesting. Table 4.1 below provides a short overview of the signers that were chosen for the current study as well as information about the age of acquisition of ISL and the languages used for family communication (taken from Mohr 2012:193).

Table 4.1 Signers chosen for the analysis of mouth actions in ISL

	Age group	**Age of sign language acquisition**	**Language of communication with family**
Caroline	1	6 years	English
Eilish	3	18 years	family signs
Fergus D.	2	2–3 years	ISL
Fergus M.	2	6 years	English, fingerspelling
Kevin	3	7 years	double handed alphabet (BSL manual alphabet)
Laurence	1	25 years	ABC, letters
Marian	3	unknown (has deaf brothers)	gestures
Michelle	2	10 years	English, gestures
Noeleen	2	12 years	English
Peter	3	7 years	family signs, written notes, BSL manual alphabet
Sarah Jane	1	birth	ISL, English
Sean	1	birth	ISL, family signs

In order to be able to analyze mouth actions in terms of word class, I added a word class tier. In this tier I established a word class for every lexical gloss that was annotated, leaving out gestures. A problematic issue in this context was to decide whether a gesture was an ad-hoc gesture and non-conventionalized, i.e. non-lexicalized, or if it was a gesture that, although not a sign language sign, is conventionalized and known throughout the whole ISL community. This point was crucial for the establishment of syntactic slots. Some of the non-conventionalized gestures substituted the predicate of a sentence or even made up the whole utterance. While this is a ubiquitous phenomenon in spontaneous speech as well (cf. for example a doctor telling his nurse to hand him a scalpel by simply saying "Scalpel!" and opening his hand), it hampered the determination of syntactic slots. All utterances including non-conventionalized gestures were excluded from the first step of the analysis aiming at establishing the basic syntactic categories of ISL.[42] The frequency of non-conventionalized gestures seems to depend on several factors such as linguistic competence. Good sign language skills seem to limit the excessive use of gestures (signers from Deaf families generally used fewer gestures than signers from hearing families) and the degree of involvement (e.g. Chafe 1982; Tannen 1985). However, the investigation of involvement and detachment has not been researched for sign languages so far and was not one of the central issues of this book. A few examples of non-conventionalized gestures in the data are shown below. Examples (1) and (2) show sentences that are completely predicateless as far as lexical signs are concerned, while in example (3) the whole utterance consists of one gesture.[43]

(1) INDEX+me INDEX+fl INDEX+me 'sure just leave it for now'
'I thought I would just leave it for now.'

(2) OKAY 'let's go then' 'sauntering over' 'thumbs up'
'So we said "okay, let's go then" and [and sauntered over] to the boy with the motorbike.'

(3) 'all done'
'That's all.'

Gestures were also not allocated a word class on the word class tier. They were simply classified as "gesture".

Another methodological problem was the establishment of sentence boundaries. The same issue has been raised by other researchers (Erlenkamp 2000, for example), who mention that this is a common problem when analyzing spontaneous speech. Sometimes participants would stop and correct mistakes they made or leave sentences unfinished. These unfinished sentences could not be considered for my analysis either.

Finally, I distinguished mouthings from mouth gestures for my investigation although I did not split the mouthing tier from the ELAN files in two as I did not want to change the original annotations made by the native speakers. I made the distinction between mouthings and mouth gestures in statistical analyses thus counting instances like the manual sign LADDER being accompanied by a mouthed 'ladder' as mouthings and instances like the manual sign SHAPE-OF-ENGINE accompanied by an 'open, clenched teeth' mouth as mouth gestures.

4.2. Categorization of Mouth Actions in the SOI Data

In the following, a categorization of the mouth actions that were found in the SOI is provided. For mouth gestures this has been done by other researchers for other sign languages. The applicability of these classifications to ISL will be discussed in section 4.2.2.

A categorization of mouthings was usually not carried out for other sign languages. Only recently, Bank et al. (2011:256) suggested a classification of mouthings into standard mouthings, mouthings variants and overlaps in NGT. Regarding the form and semantics of the manual-mouthing relationships, this seemed necessary for ISL as well. While a relation of formal and semantic congruence[44] holds true for many of the mouthings observed, others were divergent from the manual sign itself or the concept expressed by the latter. In Mohr (2012:197) I hence propose a classification of ISL mouthings into 6 types according to formal[45] and semantic criteria. This typology is taken up in 4.2.1 and explained in further detail.

The different types of mouthings and mouth gestures are discussed qualitatively in the next two sections while they are evaluated quantitatively with respect to linguistic and sociolinguistic factors in chapters 5 and 6.

4.2.1. Mouthings

Concerning the quality of mouthings, there are many different possibilities of combinations with manuals. Generally, there are three larger categories describing the match of mouthing and manual sign when referring to the parameters mentioned in the previous section.

1. One-to-one matches of mouthings and manual signs. (Standard mouthings in Bank et al.'s classification.)
2. Mouthings and manuals that do not match 100% but are related formally or semantically. (Mouthings variants in Bank et al.'s classification.)
3. Mouthings and manuals that seem not to be related neither formally nor semantically. (A special kind of mouthing variants in Bank et al.' classification.)

An example of the first large category mentioned above, are semantic and formal one-to-one matches of mouthings and manual signs or the canonical gloss[46] usually associated with a sign, as e.g. KNOW and "know", LEARN and "learn", DRINK and "drink", DEAD and "dead", HAPPY and "happy", FOOL and “fool”, CHAIR and “chair”, MONTH and “month” or BALL and “ball”. The sign CHAIR is shown in figure 4.4.

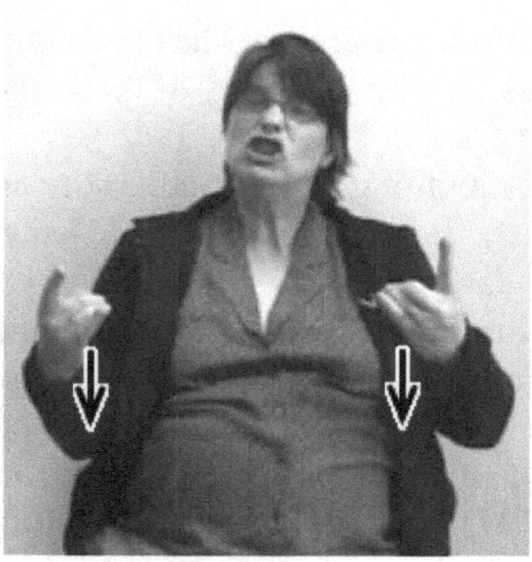

Figure 4.4 TYPE 1 mouthing

It also seems noteworthy that this kind of mouthing is the most common combination of mouthing and manual sign. This semantic redundancy is also mentioned in other studies (e.g. Plaza Pust 2005). Subsequently, this kind of matching is called **TYPE 1**.

A mouthed word and a manual or gloss might only be semantically related while they are not alike in form, as mentioned by Boyes Braem (2001) for her DSGS data. Instances of this are BIG and “massive”, FALSE and “fake”, CUP-OF-TEA and “cappuccino”, MOTORBIKE and “scooter”, JOB and “work” or LIKE and “love”. This relation of manual sign and mouthing is classified as **TYPE 2**. The sign CUP-OF-TEA accompanied by the mouthing “cappuccino” is shown in 4.5.

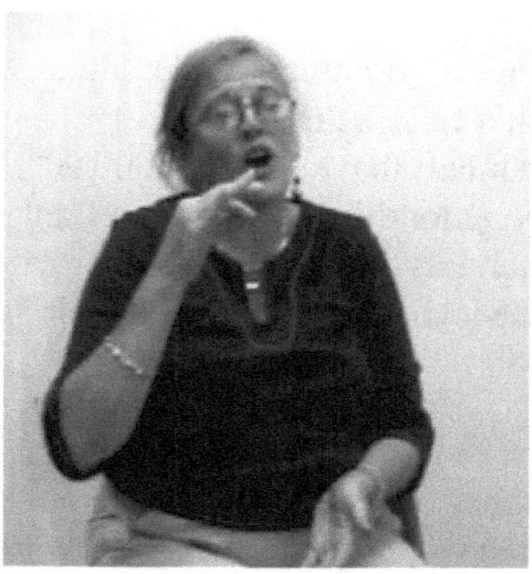

Figure 4.5 TYPE 2 mouthing

Although the next type is very similar to TYPE 2 (semantically similar but formally different mouthings) with respect to its semantics, it is different in form, which is why I decided to assign it a category of its own. Many verbs that have to be translated as prepositional verbs are only accompanied by the blank mouthed verb as in GO-IN/GO-OFF and "go". Further examples are PACKING-UP and "pack", THROW-OUT accompanied by a mouthed "throw" or LOOK-UP/LOOK-FOR and "look". THROW-OUT combined with "throw" can be seen below.

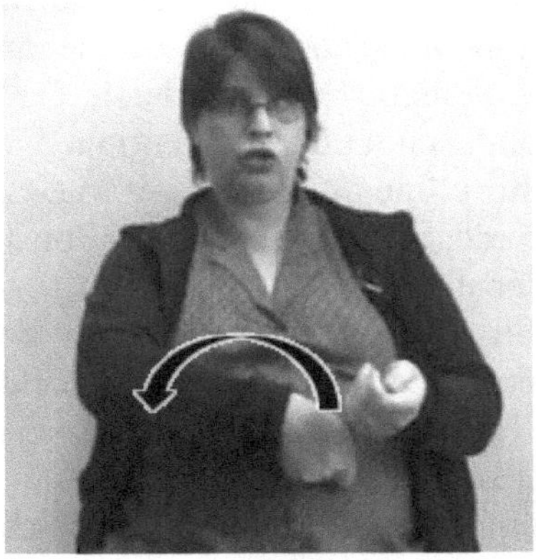

Figure 4.6 TYPE 3a mouthing

Similar instances can be found especially with incorporated elements and classifier constructions. Thus, THROW-BALL-UP might only be accompanied by "throw" and SCORE-IN-BASKETBALLNET by "scored", PUT-SMALL-OBJECT-IN-ENGINE and "put in", MEET-PERSON++ and "meet, meet, meet", TANK-FILLS-UP and "fill" or JUMP-OVER-OBJECT and "jump". The manual MEET-PERSON++ accompanied by "meet" is depicted in figure 4.7.

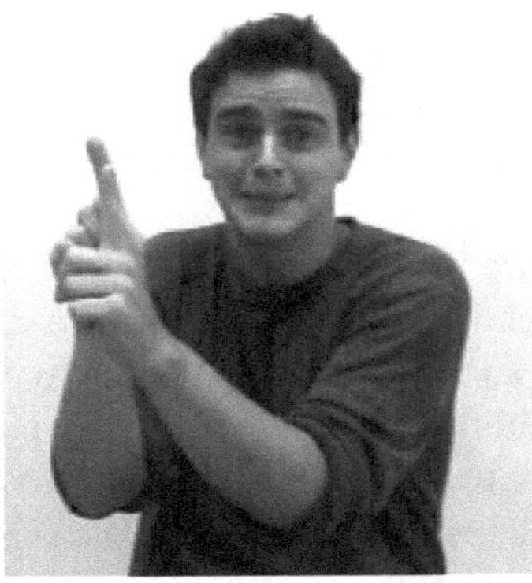

Figure 4.7 TYPE 3b mouthing

This kind of combination of manual signs and mouthings might hint at the fact that the verb is the most salient part of this construction. However, instances where only the noun in the construction is mouthed, could be observed as well. Examples of this kind are HOLD-OBJECT-AND-HANDBAG accompanied by a mouthed “bag”. These instances are rarer than the version mentioned above. In 57% (= 40 items) of these cases, the manual was accompanied by the verb only, while in 43% (= 30 items) of all cases, the construction was combined with either the object that is concerned or a preposition. Why these mouthings behave differently, cannot clearly be determined at this point. The nature of the mouthings in the latter constructions hints at pragmatic reasons though. Frequently, the object that is expressed on the mouth is not directly mentioned in the manual but rather relates to the overall story line as in 2x-CL-V EYE-GAZE-MEET and “Sarah Jane”. This defies the idea of saliency of the construction and hints at a discourse-related explanation.

The existence of this mouthing type actually contradicts claims from earlier studies (Hohenberger & Happ 2001; Plaza Pust 2005) that information on inflecting verbs or classifiers cannot be expressed by lexical mouthings. Referring to the ISL data, this statement has to be revised stating that although it is certainly rare that information on classifiers is expressed on the mouth, it is possible to do so.

As the two types of combinations treated in this paragraph are so similar in that the mouthing consists of the apparently most salient element shown by the manual sign, I have decided to put them into the same category. The constructions involving English prepositional verbs are classified as **TYPE 3a** while the classifier constructions are categorized as **TYPE 3b**. The main reason for classifying them as one type only is the way the unique means of sign languages are used in the manual signs in both cases. Consequently, the use of space is meaning distinguishing in TYPE 3a. For example THROW-OUT can be distinguished from THROW because the movement path of the signs is usually different. In TYPE 3b, the use of sign language unique classifier constructions (in space) defines the combination.[47]

An interesting case are inflected mouthings accompanying verbs such as LEAVE and “left”, FIND and “found” or SAY and “said”, THINK and “thought”, WIN and “won”, WANT and “wants” or SEE and “will see”. Moreover, plural forms of nouns are sometimes found in mouthings. Examples of this are POINT and “points”, HOLIDAY and “holidays”, PHOTOGRAPH and “photos”. This kind of mouthings constitutes **TYPE 4**. The sign PHOTOGRAPH accompanied by the mouthing “photos” can be seen in figure 4.8.

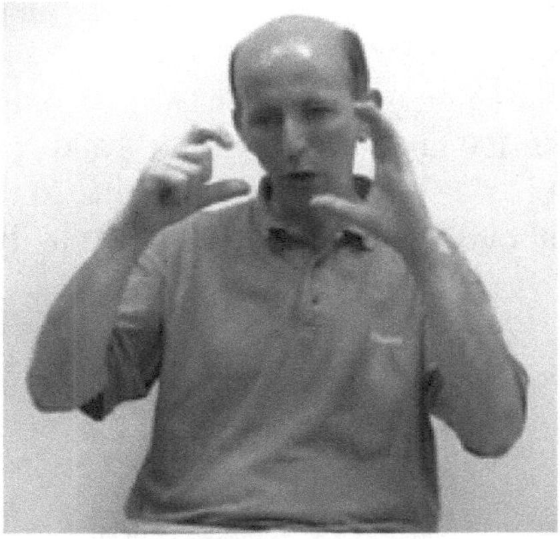

Figure 4.8 TYPE 4 mouthing

The phenomenon described above has also been observed for other sign languages such as ASL or NGT (e.g. Emmorey et al. 2005; Baker & van den Bogaerde 2008). In these studies, however, it was attributed to bimodal code-blending and ultimately a mechanism to ensure congruency between the sign language and the spoken language element on a morphological level. While the sign language verb might not be marked with a morphological marker on the verb itself, the whole sentence might be marked for past (or future) tense. In English, the morphological marker is on the verb so that at a first glance, the manual and the mouthing seem to be less congruent, while after a close analysis using the inflected English verb form, they become congruent. Emmorey et al. (2005) mention that this mechanism is especially easily applied to verbs as sign language verbs are produced with their own morphology while the spoken language verbs can show tense inflections at the same time. Moreover, the spoken and the signed language material are produced by different articulators. The two morphological systems hence do not impede each other. They claim that aspectual marking of the iterative in ASL that is often matched with repetitions of the English verb is similar. Emmorey and colleagues also claim that this is not as easily possible with nouns while Baker and van den Bogaerde (2008) found a lot of these instances in their study. As mentioned earlier, some instances concerning nouns were found in the SOI. However, they were more frequent in verbs.

While the explanation of the creation of congruency seems plausible concerning the ISL data, I would want to isolate it from its code-blending context. The context of data collection for the SOI was completely different from the contexts of the data in the other studies cited above. Consequently, it seems plausible that the signers either deliberately or unconsciously want to create semantic and morphological congruence although not in a code-blending setting.[48]

Cases of reduced mouthings of the type PART accompanied by "p-", BRILLIANT and "brill-", FINISH and "fsh", PRACTICE and "pra-pra-", LANGUAGE and "l-" or WANT and "wa-" also occurred, similar to the Bank et al. (2011) study. BRILLIANT combined with "brill-" is shown in figure 4.9.

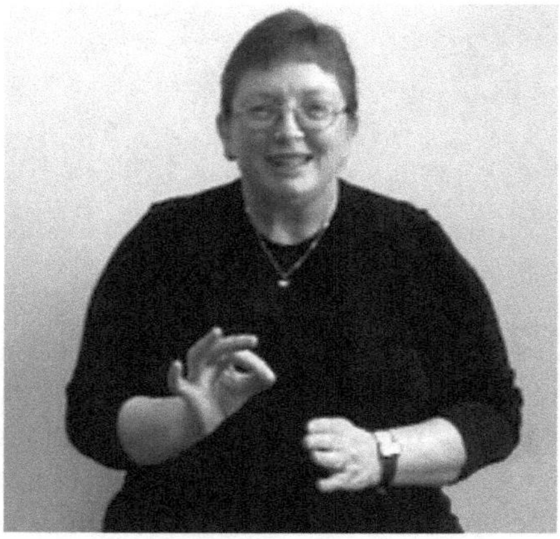

Figure 4.9 TYPE 5 mouthing

However, these instances were rather rare in the annotations in general. This might be due to the fact that transcriptions were made by deaf researchers living in Ireland. These researchers are likely to be phonologically biased, because they are surrounded by spoken English in their everyday lives. This problem was already addressed in chapter 3.2.3, where it was connected to the McGurk effect. Furthermore, the annotators might have transcribed what they think should be there (as far as they are concerned) but not what was actually uttered. Generally, the deaf researchers transcribed full mouthings, also in cases that seem debatable to me (a non-native speaker of English). This aspect of the transcription might require re-evaluation.[49] This analysis was made on the basis of the existing annotations, as I relied on the native speakers' judgments. However, I have re-analyzed the data with respect to this issue and it can be stated that the frequency of this type of mouthings is sufficient in order to form a separate type. Reduced mouthings constitute **TYPE 5** combinations.

Finally, there are mouthings that seem not to match the manual sign at all. An example of this apparent mismatch is the manual sign KNOW and the mouthing "hope" which is not directly semantically or in any other way related to the manual sign. This phenomenon can be explained by several different scenarios. Sometimes the mouthing might add an additional nuance of meaning to the manual sign, in other cases, these mouthings may be spread mouthings from a neighbouring sign and finally, the manual signs of both concepts might be metalinguistic remarks. I have categorized these kinds of mouthings as general **TYPE 6**, with more fine-grained distinctions into **TYPE 6a, b, c**.

Examples of the first case (**TYPE 6a**), a mouthing adding an additional nuance of meaning, are STRIPES-ON-TOP-OF-SHOES combined with "brown, beige", BELIEVE accompanied by a mouthed "can't", KNOW and "didn't", ENGINE and "turn on there", SIGNING and "go on" or REDUCE modified in one case by "lucky" and in another by "cheap". STRIPES-ON-TOP-OF-SHOES combined with "brown, beige" can be seen below.[50]

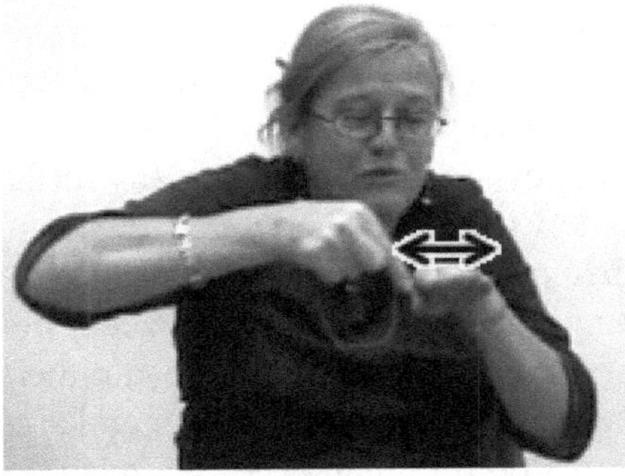

Figure 4.10 TYPE 6a mouthing

When analyzing some of the examples further, the functions of the mouthings in these seemingly random combinations become apparent. The whole sentence involving STRIPES-ON-TOP-OF-SHOES can be seen in (4).

	"shoes"	closed, round "ao"	closed, stretched "ao"	open, stretched___"brown"
(4)	SHOES	POINTED-SHOES	EXPENSIVE	STRIPES-ON-TOP-OF-SHOES
	"BEIGE"			

*b.i.

'The shoes were pointed shoes, expensive and had brown (and) beige stripes on top.'

"Brown, beige" further defines the stripes that are mentioned in the manual sign in the first example. In the combination of the manual sign REDUCE and "cheap"/"lucky", the manual is further defined by stating that something became cheap because of the reduced price and that this was a lucky circumstance. The example of the sign STRIPES-ON-TOP-OF-SHOES is similar to cases found for Norwegian Sign Language by Vogt-Svendsen (2001) which she called simultaneous compound signs (cf. chapter 3.2.3). Just as "rød" combined with PULLOVER adds additional meaning, "brown, beige" adds additional meaning to STRIPES-ON-TOP-OF-SHOES. This is especially interesting, since the mouthings have the status of independent lexemes in this construction as they carry independent meaning. As their meaning is not expressed in any manual sign, the importance of the mouthings is emphasized. Thus, the term "simultaneous compounds" seems appropriate and suggests the existence of this construction in ISL.

In the example of the manual REDUCE accompanied by either "lucky" or "cheap", the mouthings actually describe the results of the action depicted by the manual sign. This is similar to the simultaneous compound construction analyzed above, although it is not exactly the same thing. While the mouthings express an independent meaning that is not expressed in any manual sign as in the case mentioned above and can thus be considered independent lexemes as well, they do not create a compound in the common sense. They do not modify the sign they are combined with any further, but rather express a state or goal achieved by the action depicted in the manual verb sign. Hence, they could be described as "simultaneous modifiers".

TYPE 6b, mouthings that spread from an adjacent sign are rather frequent. Generally, mouthings have been found to spread either rightward (progressively) or leftward (regressively). While some sign languages exhibit preferences for a certain direction (cf. chapter 3.2.4), others allow both rightward and leftward spreading. In ISL, both possibilities can be observed although rightward spreading is slightly more frequent (55.7% rightward, 44.3% leftward spreading). Firstly, a few examples of progressive spreading can be seen below.

"team"______________
(5) a. TEAM COME-TOGETHER [ISL]
'The team came together.'

"know"______
b. KNOW PERSON [ISL]
'[I] know that person.'

Regressive spreading is illustrated in the following examples.

______"Greece"
(6) a. STAY GREECE [ISL]
'[We] stayed in Greece.'

_____"house"
b. ENTER HOUSE [ISL]
'[I] entered the house.'

A supplementary note seems in order. Mouthings of type 6b are only concerned with one of the manuals involved in the spreading, i.e. the manual that is not the "source" of the spread mouthing. In progressive spreading as in example (5a) and (5b) it is the manual following the source, in regressive spreading as in (6a) and (6b) it is the manual preceding the source. The other manual (the "source" of the mouthing) involved in these combinations usually shows a type 1 (formally and semantically congruent) mouthing combination.

Analyses for other sign languages revealed that spreading usually occurs from content to function word or that it establishes prosodic linking (e.g. Pfau 2005; 2009; Crasborn et al. 2008). This fact could also be observed for ISL, i.e. that spreading was especially frequent with pronouns/indexicals that usually do not occur with any mouth action so that the mouthing of the adjacent sign can easily spread onto the pronoun/indexical. Examples of this can be seen below. Sentence (7b) is also shown in figure 4.11 below.

________"keep"
(7) a. INDEX+me KEEP [ISL]
'I kept [...]'

"chair"________
b. CHAIR INDEX+me [ISL]
'My chair.'

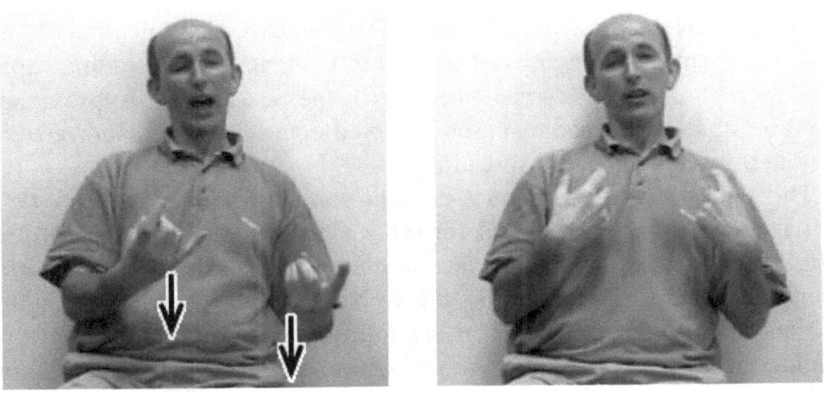

Figure 4.11 TYPE 6b mouthing

Spreading from content to function word (as in examples (7a) and (7b)) is given in the majority of the cases, i.e. that ISL seems to be word class sensitive with respect to spreading.[51] ISL seems to be similar to SSL (which also allows progressive as well as regressive spreading) in this respect.

The high frequency of instances involving pronouns and indexical signs hints at an interesting phenomenon. While it has been mentioned in the literature that pronouns often cliticize in sign languages either by phonological assimilation or by linking of the content and function word by non-manual components, these processes have not been looked at from the point of view of grammaticalization. Wilcox et al. (2010) mention two different routes of grammaticalization in sign languages, one of which involves non-manual components such as mouth or eye movements. The path of grammaticalization here is from a non-conventional gesture to prosody/intonation to grammatical morphology. The other route proposed by them involves a lexical stage, thus leading from a non-conventional gesture, to a lexical sign to a grammatical marker. It seems possible that this process is happening in ISL. The mouthings (and frequently also mouth gestures for that matter) developed from non-conventional linguistic material (gestures in Wilcox et al.' model) into lexical pronouns and might ultimately, due to the high frequency of cliticization, develop into inflectional person markers. It remains to be seen whether the end of this grammaticalization path will actually be reached; further studies in subsequent years would be necessary in order to investigate this issue.

However, some examples diverge from the abovementioned pattern, such as (5a) - (6b) where the mouthing from a content word spreads onto the adjacent content word were found as well. The hypothesis of content-to-function word spreading does not hold in these cases. Crasborn et al. (2008) observed the same phenomenon for SSL and suggested the idea of prosodic binding for these cases, as does Boyes-Braem (2001) for DSGS. While Pfau (2009:6) explicitly mentions that cases of content to content word spreading "appear rather exceptional", this does not seem to be the case for ISL. Approximately one-third of all the spreading cases observed in the analyzed data were cases of content-to-content-word spreading.

The nature of the content-to-content-word spreading cases in ISL is similar to what has been found for other sign languages such as SSL and DSGS. Hence, in example (5a), the mouthing links a subject and its verb. In example (5b), the mouthing links the verb and its object while in examples (6a) and (6b) verb and adverbial are linked by the mouthing. A prosodic binding theory thus seems very likely in these cases. Although the frequency of these instances is relatively high compared to other sign languages where they do not seem to occur at all, the frequency as compared to content-to-function word spreading in ISL is rather modest. Hence, these cases do not seem to constitute possible cases of grammaticalization although they could fit one of the two routes proposed by Wilcox et al. (2010), namely the one completely bypassing the lexical stage and having prosody/intonation as a second step.

The final case to be discussed is signs and mouthings for which no relation can be established, since the mouthing neither adds an additional nuance of meaning nor is it a spread mouthing from a neighbouring sign. This last kind of combination of manual sign and mouthing is classified as **TYPE 6c**. Examples of this kind of matching are rare but still occur as in BUS-CONDUCTOR and "whatever". This mouthing did not spread from an adjacent sign, rather, it seems to be a metalinguistic remark that does not belong to the storyline. In this particular case it also seems to be a performance phenomenon that is not used deliberately in order to fulfill a specific function.

Slightly different are combinations of the kind HOLD-OBJECT-AND-HANDBAG accompanied by the mouthings "fuck, shit". In this case the mouthings apparently reflect the signer's thoughts at this moment of the story and represent an instance of constructed action. A look at the context of the mouthing reveals this. Figure 4.12 shows the combination of HOLD-OBJECT-AND-HANDBAG and "fuck, shit".[52]

_____"for my" "garden" "bag"_______ "fuck, shit"___
(8) KEEN FOR-MY GARDEN HOLD-OBJECT-AND-HANDBAG [ISL]
'[I was] keen for my garden, but holding a handbag and another object – damn.'

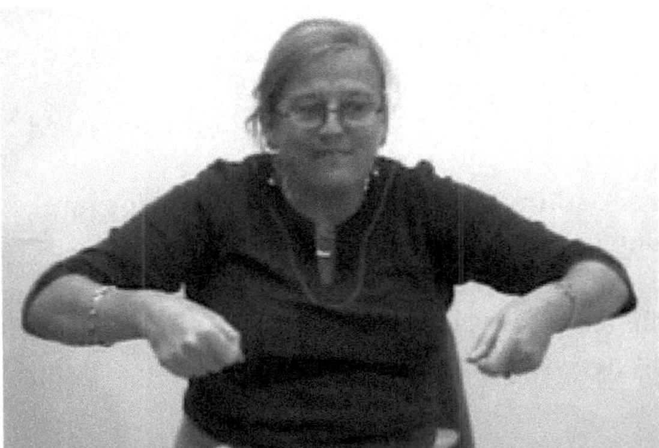

Figure 4.12 TYPE 6c mouthing

The signer was keen to take a stone she had found back home to her garden. In order to do so, she needed to put the rock in her handbag, which was too small and too full with other things. So she took some items out of the bag but the stone still did not fit. The mouthing was uttered at the moment when she realized that the stone did not fit, and she was still holding the stone and handbag. The mouthing might thus be a comment on this lack of space or the condition of holding too many objects. It is hence used deliberately, in order to convey additional information that is not expressed on the hands. However, contrasting with mouthings of the TYPE 6a (adding a nuance of meaning), it is less closely linked to one sign only but rather to the general storyline.

A similar example is the manual sign KNOW, combined with the mouthing "brown-thomas". There is no mention of the concept 'brown-thomas' in the adjacent manuals, neither in the form of a manual sign nor as a finger-spelt word. However, the sequence can be interpreted as the signer knowing Brown Thomas.[53] STORY and "continue" is another instance of this kind of combination. In this case, the manual could be related to both neighbouring signs of STORY as depicted below.

	closed, stretched up	"continue"	"go on"	
(9)	SIGNING	STORY	SIGNING	[ISL]
	'I was signing, the story had to continue, [so] I kept on signing.'			

The mouthing seems to be related to the neighbouring signs or rather to the storyline. Thus, it adds information that is related to the development of the story in general but not to the manual sign it accompanies.

This phenomenon is also exemplified in the sign INDICATOR-RISES-ON-GAUGE and the mouthing "level" in the following sign sequence:

	"level"______________________________	
(10)	INDICATOR-RISES-ON-GAUGE SURPRISE	[ISL]
	'The indicator rises on the gauge [and I am] surprised.'	

In this case, the mouthing seems to be related to the general storyline as well. Thus the meaning of the sequence is that the indicator rises on the gauge to a very high level, which surprises the acting person.

Another instance is MAN combined with the mouthing "my". Neither the left nor the right neighbouring manual sign is MY. The whole sequence is:

	____"he"	"my"	"friend"	
(11)	INDEX+fr	MAN	FRIEND	[ISL]
	'That man is my friend.'			

Again a relation to the general storyline is a possible explanation for the manual and the mouthing combining in this way. The sentence thus translates into English as "[The man] he is my friend". In this case, the mouthing seems to be a systematic means used to ensure text cohesion. This entails that the mouthing is used deliberately as it fulfills a particular function.

The final example emphasizes the point made in the previous paragraph. The manual sign DEAF and "see" were combined. The whole sentence looks as follows:

"see" closed, forward "ao"
(12) DEAF TEXT-MESSAGE [ISL]
'The deaf person sees the text message.'

Hence, the mouthing could mean that the deaf person saw the text-message. The mouthing consequently relates to the following manual sign or to the general storyline and makes the sentence more easily comprehensible.

As could be seen, there are different explanations for mismatches of mouthings and manual signs. The mouthings might add a nuance of meaning to the sign they occur with, they might be spread mouthings, a simple performance phenomenon or a systematic means of text cohesion. However, especially the explanations for TYPE 6c (metalinguistic remarks) mouthings remain speculative.

Finally, it seems noteworthy that isolated mouthings, i.e. mouthings not accompanying any manual sign, although rare, were found as well. They constitute a seventh type of mouthing, however, I have excluded them from the analysis in the subsequent chapters because I am exclusively interested in combinations and functions of manual + mouth movements.

Another combination that has not been included in the typology of mouthings discussed here is fingerspellings and mouthings. Examples are C-H-I-A-N-G-M-A-I accompanied by "Chiangmai", B-A-I-L-E-Y-S and "Baileys", W-E-X-F-O-R-D and "Wexford", N-B-A and "NBA" or C-R-E-T-E combined with "Crete". The sign C-H-I-A-N-G-M-A-I is shown in figure 4.13.[54]

The reason for excluding this type of combination from the general typology is that fingerspellings developed as contact phenomena themselves and do not constitute lexical material in the same way that manual signs do.

Summarizing, it can be stated that the overall types of mouthing-manual relations found were: one mouthing + one manual sign, two (or more) mouthings + one manual sign, a reduced mouthing + one manual sign, one mouthing + no manual sign. For the abovementioned reasons, some combinations were excluded from the final typology of mouthings and manuals

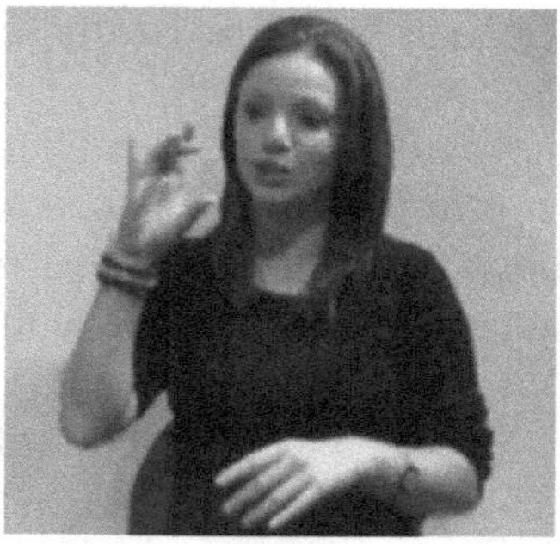

Figure 4.13 Fingerspelling and mouthing combination

here. The following combinations of mouthings were categorized for the ISL data:

TYPE 1 – One-to-one matches of mouthings and manual signs
TYPE 2 – Mouthings semantically related to the concept referred to by the manual sign
TYPE 3a –Signs that would be glossed as English prepositional verbs only accompanied by the verb referred to by the sign
TYPE 3b – Classifier constructions only accompanied by the English verb referred to by the sign
TYPE 4 – Inflected English verb form or an English plural of the conventional meaning of a sign
TYPE 5 – Reduced mouthings
TYPE 6a – Simultaneous compounds or modifiers (mouthings do not directly correspond with the lexical meaning of a manual sign)
TYPE 6b – Spread mouthings (mouthings do not directly correspond with the lexical meaning of a manual sign)
TYPE 6c – Mouthings that do not directly correspond with the lexical meaning of a manual sign they accompany but relate to the overall story

After having looked at the typology of the mouthings found in the SOI data, the following section treats the different kinds of mouth gestures that could be observed.

4.2.2. Mouth Gestures

Before actually describing the quality of the mouth gestures found in the SOI data, it should be mentioned that all mouth gestures annotated simply as "closed" were excluded from the analysis. Analyzed mouth gestures only included mouth actions that involved some kind of movement of the mouth that could not be related to any spoken English word. The mouth gestures that conformed to the abovementioned definition, were manyfold in quality. Some mouth gestures seem to be ad hoc formations and seem not to be conventionalized. This was the case if a mouth action only occurred in one signer, which hints at idiosyncratic use of the mouth gesture, or only once in general. Hence, I will mainly cite examples of mouth gestures that occurred frequently in the data, i.e. repeatedly in at least two signers. Furthermore, I will try to match the analyzed mouth gestures to the different kinds of mouth gestures mentioned in chapter 3.2.1. I utilized the labels introduced by Crasborn et al. (2008) (cf. also chapter 3) in order to differentiate the different types of mouth gestures. The three distinct types of mouth gestures found in the ISL data are hence:[55]

TYPE 1: Adverbial mouth gestures
TYPE 2: Semantically empty mouth gestures
TYPE 3: Enacting mouth gestures

The first category of mouth gestures found were **adverbial mouth gestures** (TYPE 1). An example of this is the sign that was glossed as PLAY-HARD-AGAINST-EACH-OTHER accompanied by an "open, stretched wide, jaw low, teeth clenched" mouth gesture. In this case, the clenched teeth seem to express the adverbial 'hard'. This is shown in figure 4.14 below.

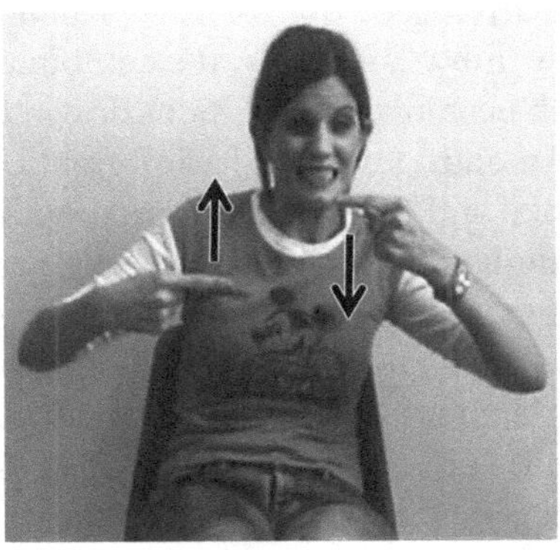

Figure 4.14 Adverbial mouth gesture 1

A similar mouth gesture could be observed in the sign PLAY-AGAINST-EACH-OTHER. In this case, the clenched teeth seem to refer to the opponent relationship that is depicted, thus emphasizing that the players did not play with each other but against each other.

Another example of this is the signs FIX-UP and REMOVE-PARTS-OF-ENGINE with a "closed, tense, bilabial" mouth gesture. This indicates that the task of fixing up that particular engine was strenuous work which could only be accomplished in a strained manner. The manual sign and mouth gesture are shown in figure 4.15 below.

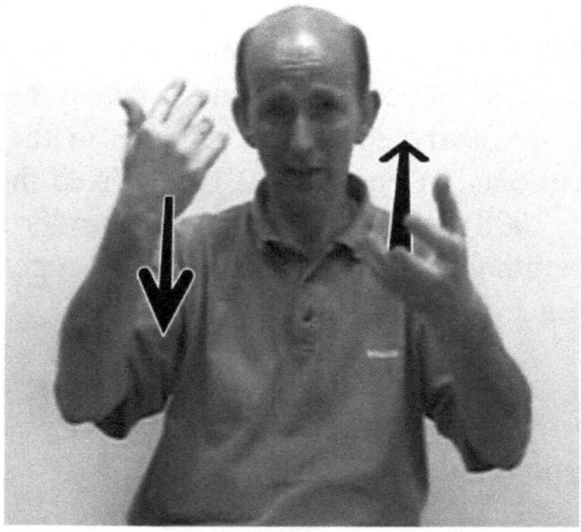

Figure 4.15 Adverbial mouth gesture 2

Another instance of an adverbial mouth gesture are the signs CAR-DRIVES-AROUND and DRIVING++ combined with the mouth gesture "ao, closed, sides down". This indicates several things. Firstly, the car does not drive very fast and secondly, the driving of the car is a prolonged action, the driving does not end after a few minutes. Finally, the combination of the manual sign ENGINE with the mouth gesture "pursed, sides down, tense" could be seen as a case of an adverbial mouth gesture. The information added to the manual sign is a mix of adverbial and adjectival information. It is supposed to depict a smoothly running engine, an engine that works perfectly, emphasized by the adjacent sign PERFECT. The mouth gesture seems to be very important in this case because the manual sign ENGINE is otherwise always accompanied by the mouthing "engine" and not by a mouth gesture. Apparently, the signer wanted to make it very clear at this point that the engine was working perfectly.[56] This is an even stronger hint at (optional) adverbial information that is added as the mouth gesture does not seem to be conventionalized for this sign.

This phenomenon is also exemplified in the combination of the manual RIDING-BOAT with a "stretched up" mouth gesture. The boat is a banana boat here and in this case, the mouth gesture expresses that the signer was happily riding the boat or having fun while riding it.

Finally, the manual sign WORK++ combined with a “closed, stretched wide, corners up” mouth gesture is an instance of an adverbial mouth gesture. The mouth gesture does not add additional meaning to the sign, it rather emphasizes that the action of working is a prolonged action and did not finish after just a few minutes. Similar cases that display the co-occurrence of the mouthing with reduplicated forms have been found with manual signs like DRIVING++ in the previous sections. WORK++ can be seen in figure 4.16.

A final example is the manual sign THROW-DOWN-SHOVEL combined with a “closed, stretched” mouth gesture. This mouth gesture adds adverbial meaning because it signifies that the shovel is thrown down in an angry manner. This claim is further supported by the subsequent sign STORM-OFF which shows that the person throwing down the shovel is indeed angry.

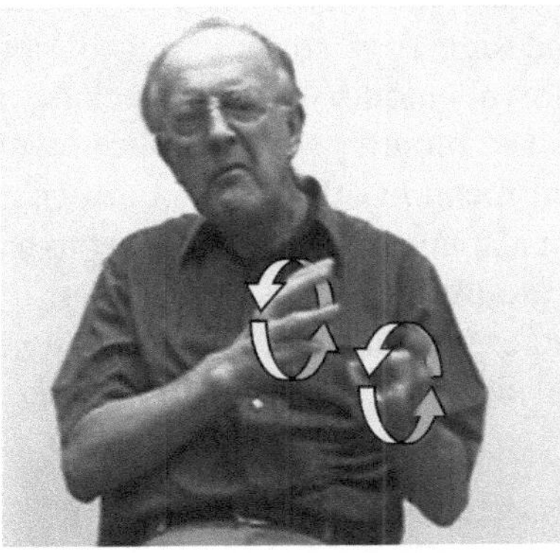

Figure 4.16 Adverbial mouth gesture 3

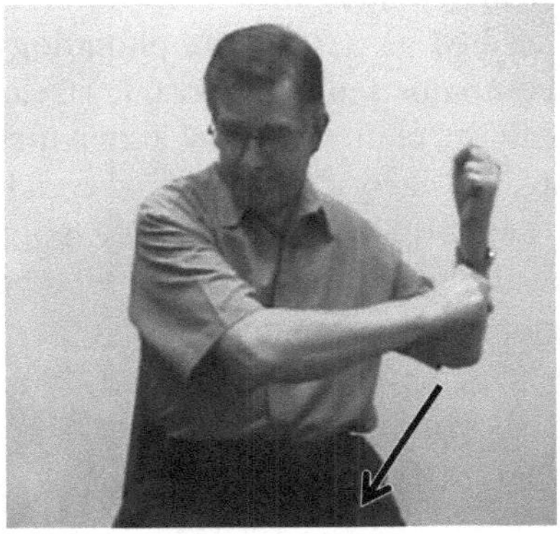

Figure 4.17 Adverbial mouth gesture 4

Another type of mouth gesture, namely **semantically empty mouth gestures** (TYPE 2), could also be observed. An example of this is the sign EXCITED accompanied by an “open, jaw low” mouth gesture (cf. figure 4.18 below).

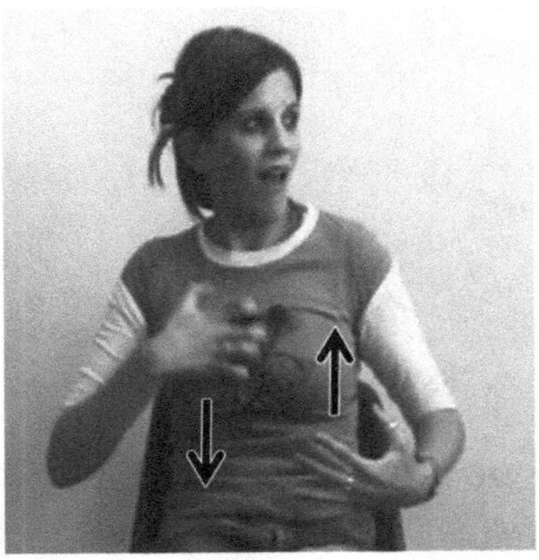

Figure 4.18 Semantically empty mouth gesture 1

In this case, the mouth gestures do not carry additional semantic information as in the case of adverbial mouth gestures. However, this mouth gesture does not seem to be obligatory for the sign, as the signer also uses the manual sign with the mouthing "excited". Thus, it does not seem to be phonologically relevant. Another example is the manual sign KEEN that was accompanied by similar mouthings of the kind "closed, forward (ao)" four times. Thus, the mouth gesture seems to be conventionalized (at least for this particular signer) as it recurs with one and the same sign. Whether the mouth gesture is actually so much conventionalized that it would be understood and used by other signers as well, could not be tested as no instances of the manual sign were found in the other signers' stories. Another example of this type of mouth gesture can be found in the sign GOOD accompanied by a "closed, stretched wide" mouth gesture. In this case, the mouth gesture could be described as part of the phonology of the sign as it could certainly not be accompanied by a "closed, stretched down" mouth gesture because this would be contrary to the sign's meaning. The mouth gesture itself, however, does not carry any adverbial or additional meaning, thus the mouth gesture was classified as semantically empty. I am also aware of the fact that in cases like these, it is hard to tell whether the mouth gesture is actually an independent mouth gesture or whether it is rather part of whole face activity that has to accompany the manual. The manual sign GOOD and the mouth gesture are shown in figure 4.19.

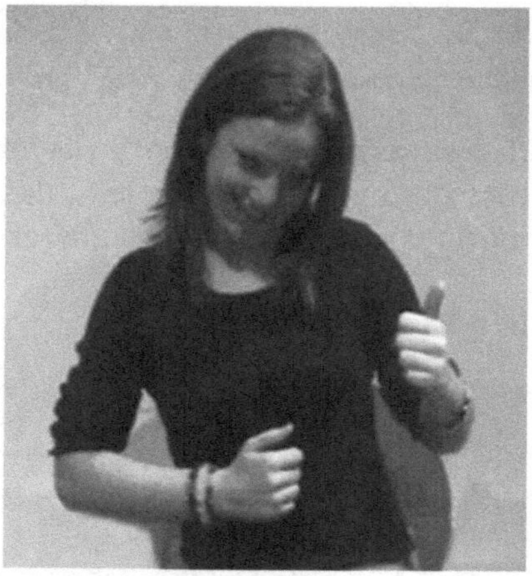

Figure 4.19 Semantically empty mouth gesture 2

The same holds true for mouth gestures occurring with the signs SURPRISE or RELIEF, for example. SURPRISE, for instance, would hardly be formed with a diverging mouth gesture unless one wanted to express a different meaning (as e.g. that something is **not** surprising). A similar example is WRONG accompanied by a "closed, stretched" mouth. With this mouth gesture, the fact that WRONG has a negative meaning, is taken up on the mouth. The sign could not be performed with a happy expression on the face and mouth. These are borderline cases of semantically empty mouth gestures and mouth gestures as part of whole face activity[57] and cannot be classified as either one or the other. Interestingly, they seem to be recurrent cross-linguistically and have been claimed to be of emotive/expressive origin (Ebbinghaus & Heßmann 1996). Semantically empty mouth gestures are also closely related to and often coincide with echo phonology. Indeed, some of the articulated elements mentioned by Woll (2001) could also be found in the ISL data. These instances include bilabial and labiodental elements, low central vowels for example. Inhalation and exhalation breath patterns could also be observed.

Another example of a semantically empty mouth gesture is the sign ENDURE combined with the mouth gesture "closed, bilabial, tense". This mouth gesture does not add adverbial or any other kind of information to the manual sign and it seems to be part of the phonology of the sign as well. It is shown in figure 4.20 below.

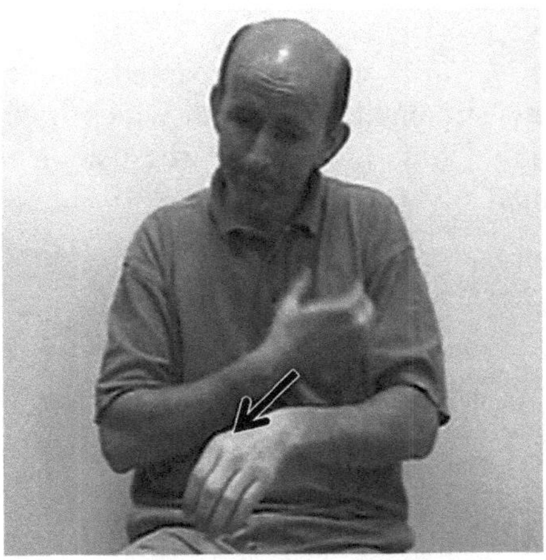

Figure 4.20 Semantically empty mouth gesture 3

Further, the manual sign CURIOUS and the mouth gesture "wrinkled nose, open, left corner up" were combined. This depicts the expression of a curious person and seems to be part of the phonology of the sign, as it could certainly not be formed with a bored expression on the face and on the mouth. As was already the case in several other instances mentioned, the activity of the mouth seems to be part of whole face activity here.

The third type of mouth gesture that was found is **enacting mouth gestures** (TYPE 3). Due to the nature of the stories that were told, several examples occurred in the women's signing. One example is the sign LICK accompanied either by a mouth gesture transcribed as "lick" or "open, stretched, jaw low, tongue 40%". In this case, the mouth gesture is clearly part of the sign, i.e. that the sign could not be formed without the mouth gesture, as is shown in figure 4.21.

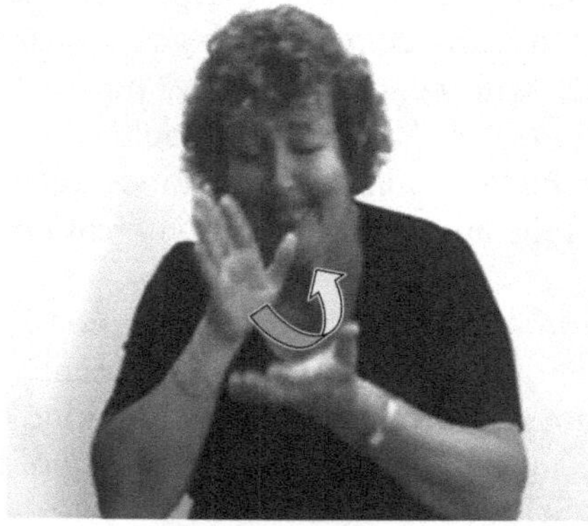

Figure 4.21 Enacting mouth gesture 1

Moreover, the sign LAUGH++ was accompanied by either an "open" mouth or an "open, jaw low, stretched up" mouth which both enact the action of laughing on the mouth. These mouth gestures also clearly depict the action depicted by the manual sign (cf. figure 4.22).

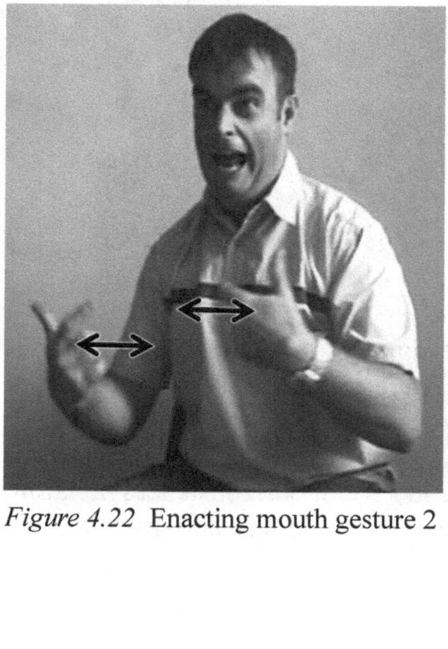

Figure 4.22 Enacting mouth gesture 2

Another example of this phenomenon is the sign CALL combined with the mouth gesture "open, jaw low". This depicts the action of calling out to another person (that is hearing). The mouth gesture actually constitutes the main sign in this case, the hands only play a minor role in forming this sign. They are partly cupped over the mouth, thus emphasizing that the action performed is directed at a certain person, as shown in figure 4.23 below.[58]

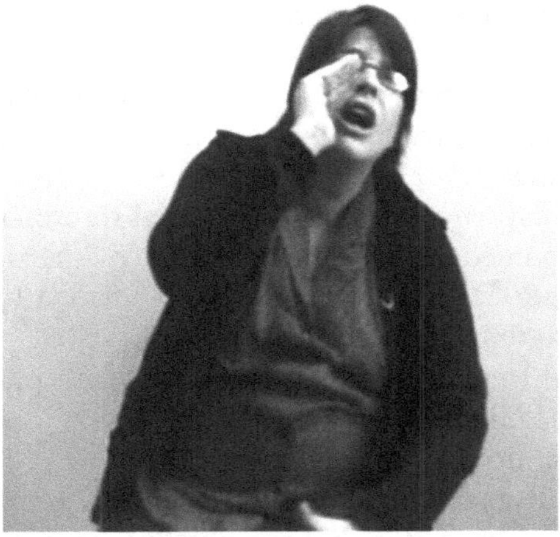

Figure 4.23 Enacting mouth gesture 3

Further, the sign CRY++ was combined with the mouth gesture "open, jaw low, tongue 10%". Just as in the other examples, the mouth reflects the action expressed by the manual sign.

As can be seen in the above classification and qualitative analysis of the mouth gestures occurring in the SOI data, no independent class of "mouth gestures as part of whole face activity" was established. This is due to the fact that it was rather difficult to classify mouth gestures as belonging to this category only. Many of the mouth gestures categorized as "semantically empty" are part of a larger whole face activity that is inherently linked to the manual sign and its phonology. Moreover, some of the signs classified as enacting mouth gestures form part of the activity of the whole face (CRY, for example). Further, many of these mouth gestures are rather expressions of emotions than a linguistic means of communication. This issue was already commented on in section 3.2.1. Consequently, I think it impossible to set up a fourth category of mouth gestures. A similar approach was taken by Lewin and Schembri (2009), who only used the categories "adverbial, enacting mouth gestures" and "echo phonology".

4.2.3. Mouth Actions in the SOI at a Glance

The previous two sections provided a qualitative analysis of the two kinds of mouth actions found in the SOI, namely mouthings and mouth gestures. Furthermore, several subcategories of the broader classes mouthings and mouth gestures were established, which seemed necessary given the large variety of different types especially in the mouthings class. Thus, six different types of mouthings (based on Mohr 2012:197) relevant for the current analysis were established. They are listed below.

TYPE 1 – One-to-one matches of mouthings and manual signs
TYPE 2 – Mouthings semantically related to the concept referred to by the manual sign
TYPE 3a – Signs that would be glossed as English prepositional verbs only accompanied by the verb referred to by the sign
TYPE 3b – Classifier constructions only accompanied by the English verb referred to by the sign
TYPE 4 – Inflected English verb form or an English plural of the conventional meaning of a sign
TYPE 5 – Reduced mouthings
TYPE 6a – Simultaneous compounds or modifiers (mouthings do not directly correspond with the lexical meaning of a manual sign)
TYPE 6b – Spread mouthings (mouthings do not directly correspond with the lexical meaning of a manual sign)
TYPE 6c – Mouthings that do not directly correspond with the lexical meaning of a manual sign they accompany but relate to the overall story

Two types of mouthings were left out of the above list: isolated mouthings, i.e. mouthings that do not accompany any manual sign and mouthings accompanying a fingerspelt sign. The two main reasons for not including them in this typology of mouthings are a) that instances of isolated mouthings were rather rare, and b) that the above classification is concerned with combinations of manual signs and mouthings only, while neither isolated mouthings nor fingerspelt signs involve manual signs in the usual sense.

Concerning the second larger category of mouth actions, namely mouth gestures, the classification applied to NGT, SSL and BSL by Crasborn et al. (2008) was utilized. For reasons mentioned in section 4.2.2, only three of the four categories mentioned in this paper were applied to the ISL data. Accordingly, three subclasses of mouth gestures were identified:

TYPE 1 – Adverbial mouth gestures
TYPE 2 – Semantically empty mouth gestures
TYPE 3 – Enacting mouth gestures

After the qualitative analysis of mouth actions in the data, the next two chapters will provide a quantitative analysis of mouth actions in the SOI data. In the following chapter, the data will be investigated with respect to sociolinguistic factors, such as gender and age, while in chapter 6, an analysis referring to the linguistic factor word class will be conducted.

Chapter 5
Mouth Actions in ISL – Sociolinguistic Factors

In this chapter, current findings on sociolinguistic factors influencing mouth actions in ISL with respect to the Signs of Ireland Corpus are discussed. Suggestions from earlier works such as Ó Baoill and Matthews (2000) will be considered for the analysis.

To this end, the chapter is subdivided into three subchapters. The first subchapter outlines research questions and hypotheses regarding the sociolinguistic factors gender and age. Afterwards, mouth actions with respect to gender are elaborated on and subsequently, in the last subchapter, the sociolinguistic factors gender and age are combined and the results of the whole chapter are discussed.

5.1. Research Questions and Hypotheses

The current study is the first to investigate mouth actions in ISL empirically and systematically. Although mouth actions are mentioned by most researchers, these claims are often based on their own language competence instead of empirical research. Thus, utterances remain rather vague as was already mentioned previously. The aim of the current study is hence to investigate whether mouth actions in ISL are used systematically and whether certain patterns with regard to linguistic and sociolinguistic factors can be observed.

The sociolinguistic factors that possibly play a role with respect to mouth actions are gender and age. Age is accredited as an important factor in the literature as well, as Ó Baoill and Matthews (2000:10) claim: "Older deaf people [...] use no lip-patterns [mouthings] to accompany their meanings [...]" and "Younger deaf people in Ireland [...] articulate these meanings [...] with the addition of English influenced lip-patterns [mouthings]". A signer's age might especially influence his/her mouthing behaviour, as this is largely language contact induced (cf. chapter 3.2.3). This language contact was enforced in deaf schools, to which the oralist method (cf. chapter 2.2) was introduced at different times. Consequently, I hypothesize that a signer's age has an impact on his/her mouth action behavior in that older signers who were educated before the introduction of oralism use less mouthings than younger signers who were educated in the oralist method. Gender, as mentioned in chapters 2.1 and 2.2, is an important factor not only concerning the lexical level but also other linguistic levels such as that of discourse in ISL. Therefore, I hypothesize a signer's sex to have a considerable impact on his/her mouth action behavior, especially because oralism was introduced at different times to the boys' and girls' school. With respect to mouth gestures, age and gender are not expected to have any effect.

5.2. Mouth Actions and Gender

As was already mentioned previously, gender variation plays an important role in ISL not only on the lexical level. Other researchers like Ó Baoill and Matthews (2000) already anticipated that gender variation has to exist with respect to mouth actions in ISL. In the following, this claim will be investigated empirically for the SOI data, drawing on preliminary results that were presented in Mohr (2012). As a detailed qualitative analysis of mouth actions was provided in chapter 4, the discussion in the next sections will be mainly quantitative. I will start with an evaluation of mouth actions in women, followed by an analysis for the men. The last section provides a summary of the obtained results in the form of a comparison of the two groups.

5.2.1. Mouth Actions in Women

Irrespective of age groups, the category mouthings is the largest category concerning the women's mouth actions. In 62% (606) of the cases, a mouthing accompanies their manual signs. Mouth gestures occur less frequently, only 17.9% (175) of their manual signs are accompanied by a mouth gesture. 20.1% (197) of all manual signs are not accompanied by any mouth action at all. The use of mouthings varies between individual signers. Hence, the frequency of mouthings amounts to 86.8% (99) in one woman, while it is considerably lower in another one 36.6% (83). This is shown in more detail in table 5.1.

Regarding the different types of mouthings in the women, TYPE 1 (formally and semantically congruent) mouthings were the most frequent type in all women. However, with respect to the other types of mouthings that occur in individual signers, the female group is quite heterogeneous. This is exemplified by TYPE 4 (inflected English) mouthings. While some women make extensive use of inflected English mouthings, others rarely use them at all. This might be due to differences in oral training that the signers received.

Table 5.1 Mouthings in women

	No. of signs	No. of mouthings	No. of mouth gestures	No mouth action
Caroline	114	99 (86.8%)	5 (4.4%)	10 (8.8%)
Eilish	103	59 (57.3%)	25 (24.3%)	19 (18.4%)
Marian	294	211 (71.8%)	79 (26.9%)	4 (1.4%)
Michelle	227	83 (36.6%)	29 (12.8%)	115 (50.7%)
Noeleen	136	91 (66.9%)	7 (5.1%)	38 (27.9%)
Sarah Jane	104	63 (60.6%)	30 (28.8%)	11 (10.6%)
Total	978	606 (62.0%)	175 (17.9%)	197 (20.1%)

Concerning the spreading behaviour of mouthings in the women's signing (TYPE 6b, spread mouthings), both directions, i.e. rightward and leftward spreading, occur. However, although both directions are possible, rightward spreading is more frequent in the data than leftward spreading. The ratio is 58% (29) rightward to 42% (21) leftward.

Another issue refers to TYPE 6 mouthings. Generally, they (TYPEs 6a-c mouthings) occur relatively frequently in one signer while they do not occur at all in others. Thus, these mouthings are by no means a phenomenon that is conventionalized in any way. An interesting case is one particular signer who produced extraordinarily many mouthings that did not fit the manual sign. In her case, the manual signs of both concepts were indeed phonologically related (LADDER and BIKE which are distinguished by different handshapes and slightly different movements), however, she produced the mouthing mistakes deliberately. Her personal story was about a misunderstanding between her and her daughter who continually produced the sign LADDER while actually meaning BIKE and using the mouthing "bike", too. Apparently, the daughter's mouthings did not disambiguate the situation.[59] The use of mouthings in this way has also been reported by Boyes Braem (2001) who referred to it as "constructed speaking", i.e. the imitation of hearing people's speech. An example of this mismatch between sign and mouthing in the SOI can be seen in figure 5.1.

Finally, instances of mouthings occurring without a sign that have been reported by other researchers for other sign languages, could also be found in the ISL data. However, these instances were extremely rare and are definitely an exception from the normal pattern of matching manual signs and mouthings.

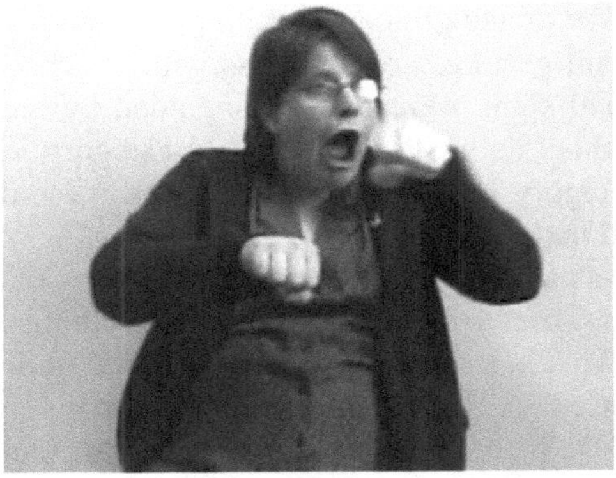

Figure 5.1 Mismatch of the manual sign bicycle and the mouthing "ladder"

For the second part of this discussion, I now want to turn to mouth gestures. Just as the frequency of mouthing varies between individual signers, it varies with respect to mouth gestures. Thus, one woman uses 28.8% (30) mouth gestures while another one uses only 4.4% (5) with her signing. This difference will also be discussed in detail in section 5.2.3.

All three different kinds of mouth gestures occurred in the women's signing. As examples of the types of mouth gestures were provided in section 4.2.2, I only want to mention some often recurring mouth gestures which would need to be classified as different types of mouth gestures according to the manual sign they accompany. Examples of these mouth gestures are "closed, stretched up/down" and "open, stretched up/down". The signs they occurred with varied a lot, thus they accompanied verbs, adjectives and indexical signs alike. This implies that they are not limited to certain signs or even constitute an obligatory part of certain signs. However, it is striking that they occurred even in those women who used very few mouth gestures in general. Hence these mouth gestures might be part of the core inventory of mouth gestures of ISL.

With respect to the different types of mouth gestures, TYPE 3 (enacting mouth gestures) was less frequent than TYPEs 1 (adverbial mouth gestures) and 2 (semantically empty mouth gestures) but not significantly so.

After having discussed the occurrence of mouth actions in women, the next section analyses mouth actions in men.

5.2.2. *Mouth Actions in Men*

In contrast to the women's mouth actions investigated in the preceding section, mouthings do not constitute the largest category in the men's signing. Irrespective of age groups, mouthings are used with a frequency of 33.3% (458), mouth gestures are used less with 19.8% (272) while 46.9% (645) of all manual signs were not accompanied by any mouth action at all. It is striking that "nothing" is the largest category in the men while it is the smallest category in the women. However, these differences will be discussed in detail in section 5.2.3.

Moreover, it was mentioned that the mouth actions of the women varied considerably from signer to signer, no matter if mouthings or mouth gestures were concerned. This is a feature that is even more noticeable in the men. Thus, one signer used 76.7% (46) of mouthings with his signs, while another used only 1.3% (3). With respect to mouth gestures, one man used 39.6% (74) mouth gestures with his signs, while another only used 9.0% (21). These differences seem to be caused by age differences, which is why they will be elaborated on in section 5.3. The exact frequencies of the different kinds of mouth actions in the men are shown in table 5.2 below.

Table 5.2 Mouthings in men

	No. of signs	**No. of mouthings**	**No. of mouth gestures**	**No mouth action**
Fergus D.	523	297 (56.8%)	48 (9.2%)	178 (34.0%)
Fergus M.	233	3 (1.3%)	21 (9.0%)	209 (89.7%)
Kevin	212	41 (19.3%)	60 (28.3%)	111 (52.4%)
Laurence	187	67 (35.8%)	74 (39.6%)	46 (24.6%)
Peter	160	4 (2.5%)	59 (36.9%)	97 (60.6%)
Sean	60	46 (76.7%)	10 (16.7%)	4 (6.7%)
Total	1,375	458 (33.3%)	272 (19.8%)	645 (46.9%)

With respect to the different types of mouthings, the diversity of the different types is not as big as that observed in women. Hence, only three of the six men show a considerable variety of mouthings while the other three mainly show TYPE 1 (formally and semantically congruent) and 6b mouthings. Also, TYPEs 2 and 5 are generally rather rare in the men's signing. Nevertheless, reduced mouthings (TYPE 5) seem to be more frequent in men than in women. This is an issue to be taken up in 5.2.3.

Regarding TYPE 6b, spread mouthings, the direction of spreading is an interesting point. Both directions, i.e. rightward and leftward spreading are possible. Similar to the women, progressive spreading is more frequent than regressive spreading, however, the difference is not as pronounced as in women. In the men the ratio is 51.7% (15) progressive and 48.3% (14) regressive spreading.

Finally, it is noteworthy that isolated mouthings, i.e. mouthings not accompanying a manual sign, which were attested for the women, could also be found in male signing. However, these instances are rather rare.

After having provided a description of the mouthing behavior of the men, I will now discuss their mouth gestures. All three types of mouth gestures that were established in 4.2.2 could be observed for the men. Concerning mouth gestures, the male and the female group seem to be much more similar than with respect to mouthings.

The same often recurring mouth gestures that were mentioned for the women could also be found in the men. Examples of these mouth gestures are "closed, stretched up/down" and "open, stretched up/down". Just as reported for the women, the signs they occurred with varied a lot and they accompanied different lexical classes. Moreover, they occurred even in those men who used very few mouth gestures in general. This emphasizes the claim made in section 5.2.1 that these mouth gestures might be part of the core inventory of mouth gestures of ISL.

Similar to the mouth gestures described in 5.2.1, TYPE 3 (enacting) mouth gestures were generally less frequent than the other mouth gesture types.

In the following chapter, the results from 5.2.1 concerning the mouth action of the women and 5.2.2 concerning the mouth actions of the men will be summarized and compared.

5.2.3. Comparison of Mouth Actions in Men and Women

After a detailed analysis of both types of mouth actions in women and men separately, this section provides a short summary of the preceding ones in form of a comparison of mouth actions concerning both sexes. As was already mentioned briefly in the previous sections, mouth actions differ between men and women. This can be seen in figure 5.2.

As becomes apparent, mouth actions in men and women differ especially concerning the use of mouthings with their signs and with respect to those signs that are not accompanied by any mouth action. The category mouthing is thus almost twice as large in women as in men, while the picture is reversed for the category nothing (it is twice as large in men than in women). This shows that men use less mouth actions (irrespective of their type) in general. Furthermore, they use especially few English-related mouthings.

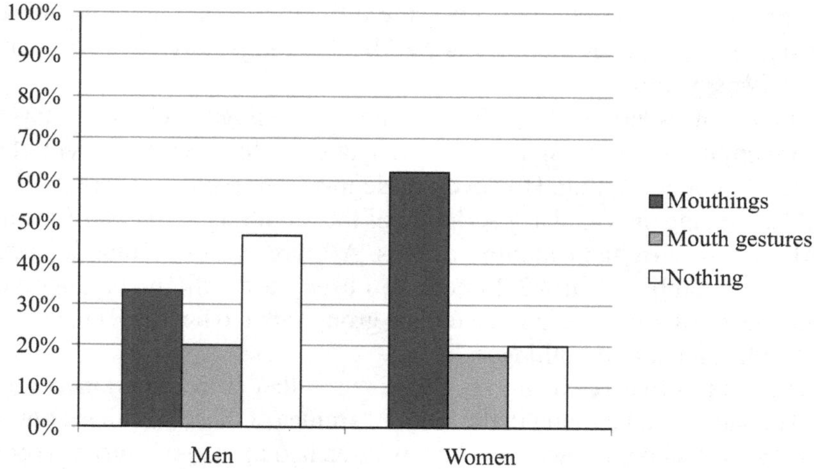

Figure 5.2 Comparison of mouth actions in men and women

It should be kept in mind, however, that the percentages for this overall comparison are not always mirrored within the two groups. Thus, there are considerable differences in mouth behaviour between individual signers, which, given the relative size of the sample, may distort the average. This is a feature that is especially prominent in the male group.

When further examining the quality of the mouth actions in men and women, both similarities and differences can be found. With respect to mouthings, all types of mouthings found in women were also found in men. The overall combinations found were: one mouthing+one manual sign, two (or more) mouthings+one manual sign, a reduced mouthing+one manual sign, one mouthing+no manual sign.

When comparing the individual types that were established in 4.2.1, it becomes clear that the men show less variety in their manual + mouthing combinations in general. A fact that becomes especially apparent is the rarity of TYPEs 4 (inflected English mouthings), 6a (simultaneous compounds/ modifiers) and c (relating to the overall story). The rarity of these types of mouthings seems interrelated as all types are concerned with mismatches of manual signs and mouthings. The discrepancies between manual and mouthing are stronger in TYPEs 6a and c, but they are still (formally) visible in TYPE 4 (inflected English) mouthings. With respect to the TYPE 4 mouthings in particular, it is logical that men show them less frequently than women, as they require a very profound knowledge of English grammar. As oralism was introduced later at the boys' school, the rarer use of "correct" English forms in mouthings seems logical. Moreover, this might be a reflection of differences in everyday use of mouthings as the social contexts in which men and women use sign language might differ.[60] Concerning the spreading behaviour of mouthings, it has already been mentioned that it is similar in men and women. Both genders show more progressive than regressive spreading, although the difference between spreading directions is larger in the women than it is in the men. This is illustrated in figure 5.3 below.

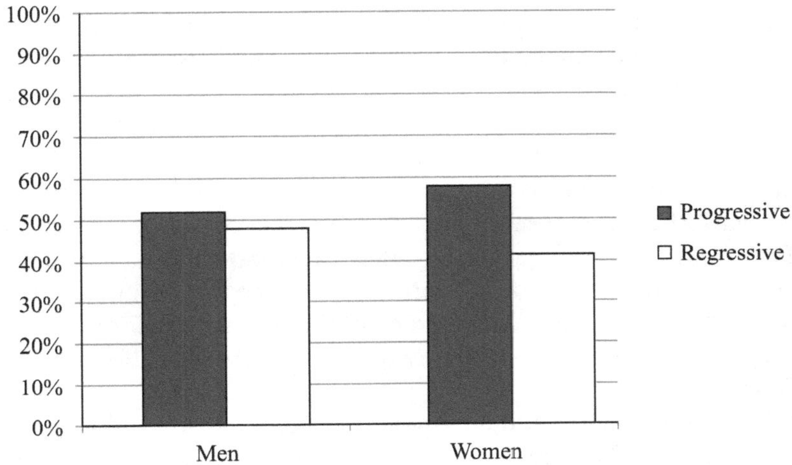

Figure 5.3 Spreading directions in men and women

In section 4.2.1 it was already mentioned that spread mouthings from content word to content word could be observed in the data. While this phenomenon occurred in both genders, it is considerably more frequent in men than it is in women: 55.2% of all spreading cases in men involved two lexical items, while it was only 18.0% in all women.[61]

With respect to mouth gestures, men and women do not behave very differently. All three types of mouth gestures from chapter 4.2.2 are found in the men's and women's signing alike. Similarly, TYPE 3 mouth gestures were least frequent in men and women.

The coincidence of the semantically empty mouth gestures found with the manual sign GOOD in both men and women hints at a shared inventory of mouth gestures for ISL. Moreover, the recurrence of certain mouth gestures like "closed, stretched up/down" or "open, stretched up/down"emphasizes this claim. Thus, in comparison to the use of mouthings, the use of mouth gestures seems to be more regular, homogeneous and more regulated within the linguistic system.

Summarizing, it can be stated that there are gender differences in mouth action behaviour in ISL, however, these only exist concerning English-based mouthings and not with respect to mouth gestures. The latter type of mouth actions seems to be fairly regulated.

5.3. Combining Two Sociolinguistic Factors – Gender and Age

As was already hinted at briefly in section 5.1, age differences play an important role with regard to mouth actions in ISL, too. These differences have been accredited in the literature (e.g. Ó Baoill & Matthews 2000), stating that older signers use less English influenced mouthings than younger signers. Although general tendencies for both sociolinguistic factors investigated could be found, the individual groups of women, men, age group 1 (younger signers), age group 2 (middle-aged signers) and age group 3 (older signers), turned out to be rather heterogeneous. A possible reason for this could be that both factors, gender and age, are interrelated and thus mutually influence each other. In order to test this, I will combine both factors in the following and analyze whether this explains some of the inconsistencies in the results obtained so far. The current chapter will thus also serve as a discussion of the previous ones.

Before elaborating on the interplay of the sociolinguistic factors gender and age, I will briefly comment on the differences in quantity and quality of the different mouth actions across the three age groups introduced in chapter 4.1. Starting with a quantitative evaluation, percentages for the different kinds of mouth movements for all three age groups are given in the below figure.

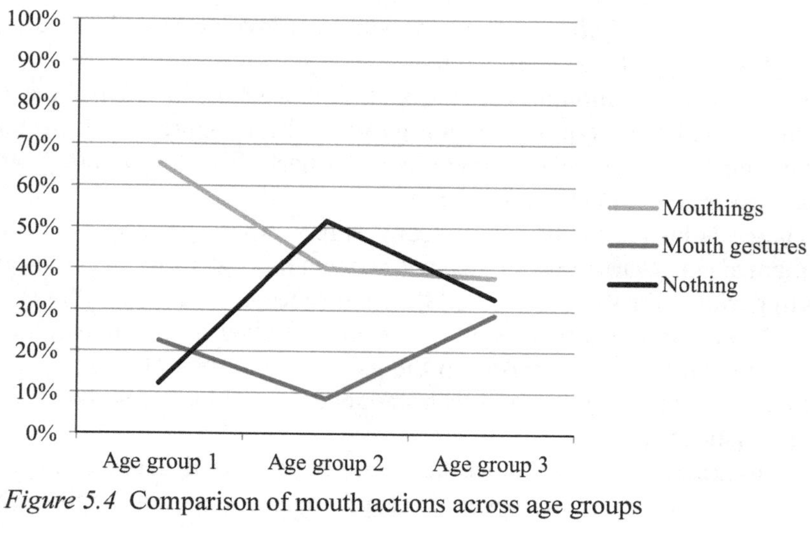

Figure 5.4 Comparison of mouth actions across age groups

The general tendency that can be inferred from this figure is that mouthings become more frequent in younger signers (age group 1) while the frequency of mouth gestures seems to decrease over the three generations. More explicitly, figure 5.4 shows that the use of mouthings increases from 37.7% in the elder signers, to 40.4% in the second age group (middle-aged signers), to 65.0% in the youngest signers. The frequency of mouth gestures however, first decreases from 29.1% in age group 3 (older signers) to 9.0% in age group 2 (middle-aged signers), only to increase to 22.4% in age group 1 (younger signers) again. It is not completely clear why the frequency of mouth gestures first decreases and then increases again. One explanation might be that the use of mouthings and the use of mouth gestures is in complementary distribution so that the increasing use of mouthings in age group 2 (middle-aged signers) causes a decrease in mouth gestures in that age group. However, an analysis of an even younger generation than the youngest signers from the SOI might shed more light on the situation. This is beyond the scope of this book and might be an issue for future researchers to tackle with new sets of data.

Finally, it can be stated that signers generally accompany more and more manual signs by some kind of mouth action as the category "nothing" first increases from age groups 3 (older signers) (33.2%) to age group 2 (middle-aged signers) (50.6%) and then reduces by more than half to 12.7% in age group 1 (younger signers).

Regarding the quality of the mouth actions, the groups are very similar, however, there are some combinations of manual sign and mouth action that occur in one group and not in another or vice versa. Generally, however, the same combinations of mouthings and manual signs that were found in men and women were found for all three age groups. Thus, the observed combinations were: one mouthing+one manual sign, two (or more) mouthings+ one manual sign, a reduced mouthing+one manual sign, one mouthing+no manual sign. While the age groups behave similarly concerning certain types of mouthings, as for example TYPE 1 (formally and semantically congruent) mouthings, other types appear more interesting as the mouthing behaviour of the groups is divergent. These are TYPE 2 (semantically similar but formally different) mouthings and especially TYPE 5 (reduced) mouthings. Hence, compared to age groups 1 (younger signers) and 3 (older signers), TYPE 2 (semantically similar but formally different) mouthings occur rarely in age group 2 (middle-aged signers). In the 36–50 year-olds' signing, the manual signs were usually combined with a mouthing that completely matches the manual sign (TYPE 1). If not, the mouthing did not match the manual sign at all; TYPE 2 (semantically similar but formally different) cases which are sort of intermediate cases thus occurred only rarely. Interestingly, the frequency of TYPE 5 (reduced) mouthings is also very divergent concerning the different age groups. They do not occur at all in the second age group (middle-aged signers), while they are relatively frequent in the third. It seems rather logical that when a certain age group uses many reduced mouthings consisting of incomplete English words, it is not very likely for them to use mouthings that contain even more information than necessarily required. This holds true for age group 3 (older signers), while it is exactly the other way around with age group 2 (middle-aged signers). They frequently express more information than necessary in their mouthings, hence reduced mouthings containing less than the complete English word are rare.

The spreading behaviour of the different age groups, although similar at a first glance, shows certain differences as well. Regarding the direction of spreading age groups 1 (younger signers) and 2 (middle-aged signers) show more progressive than regressive spreading. In contrast, age group 3 (older signers) shows more regressive spreading. Looking at the items involved in the spreading, similarities between age groups 2 (middle-aged signers) and 3 (older signers) become apparent. In these two groups, the majority of spreading cases are concerned with content to function word spreading as only one third of all cases involve content to content word spreading. In opposition to that, almost half of all spreading cases in age group 1 (younger signers) involve content to content word spreading. One possible explanation for this may be the fact that the percentage of mouthings is highest in this group which means that there are more possibilities for spreading in general.

When combining age and gender for age group 1 (younger signers) and thus breaking the age group down into a male and a female group, considerable differences especially for the category “mouthings” become apparent. While the men use 56.2% of mouthings with their signs, the women use 73.7% of mouthings. The category of “mouth gestures” also differs considerably between the men and women of the youngest generation. Hence the men use considerably more mouth gestures (28.2%) than the women (16.6%). The category “nothing” also shows noticeable differences for men and women (15.6% in men and 9.7% in women). A summary of these figures can be seen in figure 5.5.

In the second age group (middle-aged signers), differences are visible concerning all categories of mouth actions. The differences concerning the category of “mouthings” are even more pronounced than in age group 1 (younger signers). While the men use only 29.1% of mouthings with their signs, the women use 51.7%. Contrastingly, the mouth behaviour of men and

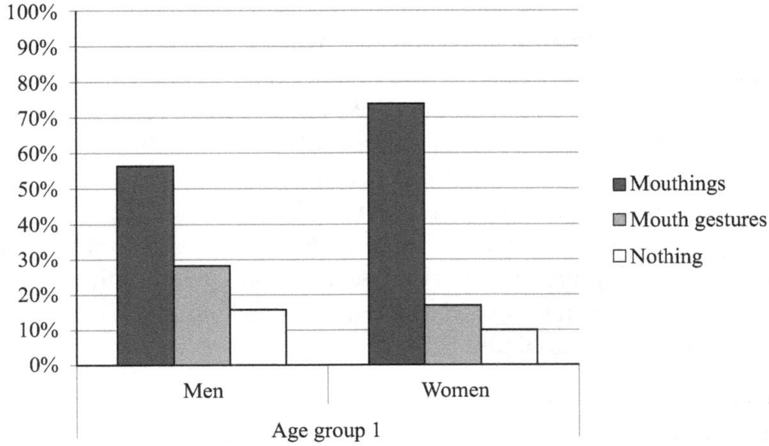

Figure 5.5 Comparison of mouth actions in men and women age group 1

women in this age group is very homogeneous with respect to the category of "mouth gestures". Both men and women use roughly 9% of mouth gestures with their signs. The category "nothing" shows a very different picture as the men do not use any mouth action with their signs in 61.8% of the cases while this figure only amounts to 39.3% in the women. A summary of this is shown in figure 5.6 below.

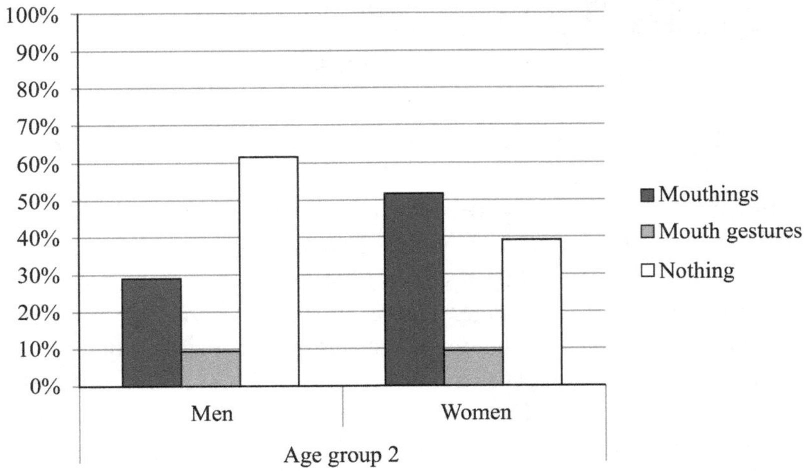

Figure 5.6 Comparison of mouth actions in men and women in age group 2

Finally, differences in mouth behaviour can also be observed in the third age group's (older signers) signing. The differences concerning the category "mouthings" are most pronounced in this age group: the men use only 10.9% of mouthings with their signs while the women use 64.5%. The category of "mouth gestures" however, shows rather similar numbers for both sexes (32.6% in men and 25.6% in women). When observing the number of signs that are not accompanied by any mouth action at all, striking differences become visible. The men do not use any mouth action at all with 56.5% of their signs which means that more than half of their signing is not accompanied by any mouth action at all. In the women, only 9.9% of all signs are not accompanied by any mouth action, so that a large part of the sign stream is accompanied by some kind of movement of the mouth. A comparison of these figures is shown in figure 5.7.

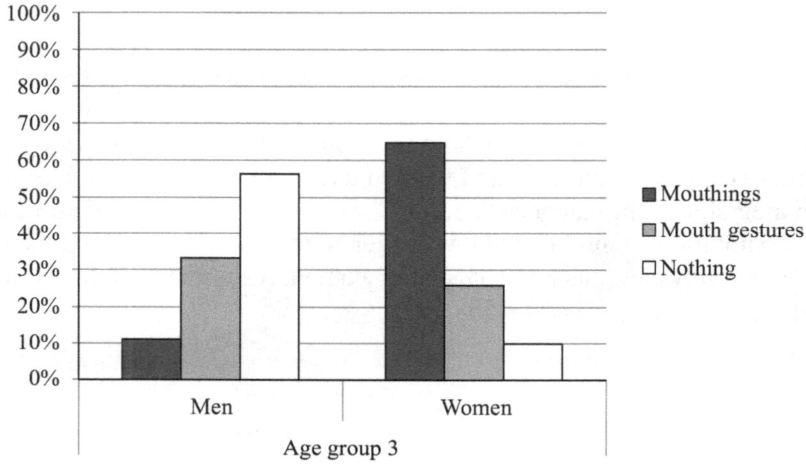

Figure 5.7 Comparison of mouth actions in men and women in age group 3

After having looked at the figures for all three age groups separately, certain trends concerning the mouth behaviour of the groups become apparent when looking at them in sum. While a general tendency towards a more frequent use of mouthings in the younger signers was already visible for the three age groups irrespective of the signers' sex, it is also visible when looking at the men's data only. However, figures are lower for the men only, starting at 10.9% in age group 3 (older signers) and ending at 56.2% in age group 1 (younger signers). Surprisingly, this upwards trend with respect to mouthings turns out to be less pronounced in the women. Figures are rather stable when comparing the three different age groups. Hence, figures start at 64.5% in age group 3 (older signers), fall to 51.7% in age group 2 (middle-aged signers) and rise again to 73.7% in age group 1 (younger signers). The women's use of mouthings is thus much more stable across apparent time, as measured by age groups than the men's concerning the category of mouthings.

Regarding the category of mouth gestures, figures for men and women are also different across the three age groups. They fall from 32.6% to 9.1% only to rise again to 28.2% in the men. In the women they fall from 25.6% to 9% and rise to 16.6% again. However, there seems to be a general downwards trend concerning the use of mouth gestures in women which is not apparent in men. A similarity of the developments is the decrease of mouth gestures in the second age group (middle-aged signers) in both sexes. This could be due to the fact that the use of mouthings and mouth gestures is interrelated, i.e. that when the use of one category is increased the use of the other category decreases.

The general trend for the use of mouth gestures across generations is slightly different from what was observed for women and men separately. The general development observed for mouth gestures across age groups irrespective of the signers' sex was a slight downward trend with an even more pronounced decrease from age group 3 (older signers) to 2 (middle-aged signers) (29.1% to 9% to 22.4%). This sudden decrease of mouth gestures in age group 2 (middle-aged signers) does not seem logical as mouth gestures are a sign language inherent feature with grammatical function and are thus necessary for the system. It might be the case that this decrease is due to the kind of stories the signers were telling. It was already mentioned that enacting mouth gestures only rarely occurred in the stories of age group 2 (middle-aged signers). This might be a possible influence on the figures.[62]

The category "nothing" seems to be the outcome of the interplay of mouthings and mouth gestures. Naturally, the category grows or diminishes influenced by the developments in the other two categories. Thus, with the increasing use of mouthings and a more or less stable use of mouth gestures in men, the occurrence of no mouthings decreases from 56.5% in age group 3 (older signers) to 15.6% in age group 1 (younger signers). The development is similar to that observed for all signers across age groups, however, figures start higher and decrease more slowly than in all signers.

The development detected for the women across the age groups is very curious. In their signing, less signs are not accompanied by any mouth action: figures increase from 9.9% in younger signers to 39.3% and rapidly decrease to 15.6% in the oldest signers again. The development is thus neither similar to the general development of the age groups nor to the development in men. This trend is however related to the figures observed for the different kinds of mouth actions. While the use of mouthings only slightly increases in the women, their use of mouth gestures decreases which results in an increase of the figures for the category nothing. A summary of the developments concerning all three categories and combining gender and age can be seen below.

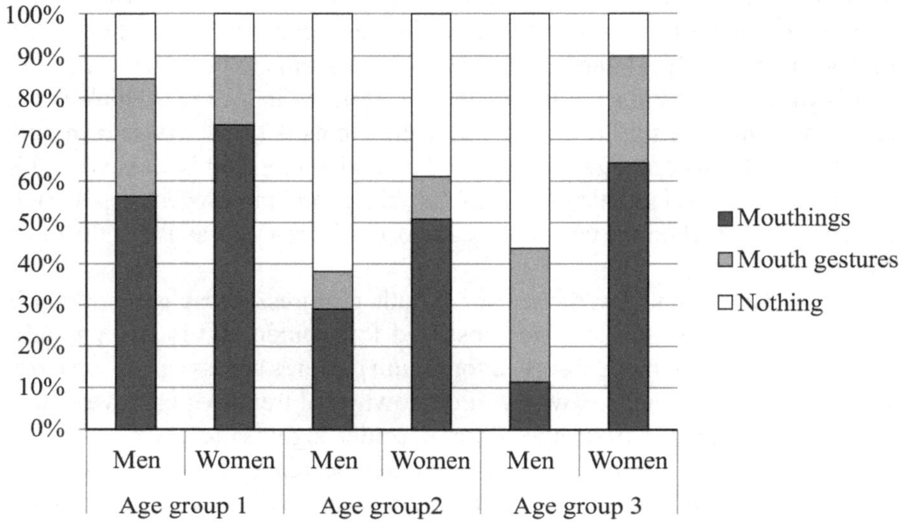

Figure 5.8 Comparison of mouth actions for all sociolinguistic factors

There are several possible reasons for the different developments concerning men and women across generations. The most plausible reason seems to be the difference in educational methods at the Cabra schools. Thus, the women who attended St. Mary's School for Deaf Girls were subjected to the oralist education method (using spoken English as the medium of instruction) much earlier than the men who attended St. Joseph's School for Deaf Boys. This is most visible in the more frequent use of language contact induced English mouthings by the women of all age groups. Even the women in the elder signers' age group already use a considerable amount of mouthings when the men only use these very infrequently. Furthermore, it is clearly observable that those younger male signers that were also subjected to the oralist education method at school use more English mouthings than the signers of the third age group (older signers). This development was also commented on in detail in Mohr (2012).

The general upwards trend towards a more frequent use of mouthings in both sexes would thus be related to the oralist education method being firmly established at both Cabra schools. The only thing that cannot be accounted for by this explanation is the difference between men and women in age group 1 (younger signers). Despite the fact that the current language policy at both schools is an oralist one, there are differences concerning the use of mouthings in male and female signers. In order to further investigate this issue, real life teaching situations and communication situations between teachers and students would have to be observed. This is beyond the scope of this book and remains a matter to be investigated by future analyses. However, it was mentioned in chapter 5.2.3 that other social factors like the social contexts in which men and women interact in their daily lives as well as differences in values men and women place on speech skills might be another influential factor.

The altogether rather stable use of mouth gestures across age groups is probably due to the fact that mouth gestures are sign language inherent. Therefore, they are a linguistic feature that is a stable (except for slight changes) part of the linguistic system. The category of mouth gestures thus seems to be the more stable of the categories of mouth actions.

This finally leads to the developments observed for the category "nothing". Across generations a downwards trend was visible which could be explained by the increasing use of mouthings across age groups. The same development holds true for the male signers, the only difference being a more pronounced development in the men. In the women, the development is the opposite: fewer signs are accompanied by any mouth action from age group 3 (older signers) to age group 1 (younger signers). This, however, could be explained by the observations made for the other categories just described.

Summing up, an account for the differences between age groups and sexes in use of the different kinds of mouth actions would entail several things. Firstly, it would mean that language contact has a major influence on sign languages and some parts of their lexicon. This can be seen in the increasing use of mouthings in ISL. Mouthings enter a sign language as cross-modal borrowings from the surrounding spoken language[63] and might ultimately acquire other, additional functions as was shown in chapter 4. They gradually become more and more established in the vocabulary of the sign language concerned. However, this fact is no particularity of sign languages but can be observed in spoken languages, too. It is merely the cross-modal component that is unique to this language contact situation.

Generally, contact phenomena range from language shift or switch to another language, integration of loan vocabulary to language change on the diachronic level (Plaza Pust 2005). In spoken languages, lexical material from another language is often borrowed as new techniques, inventions or items are borrowed from the other culture. Hence, German borrowed words such as *Toaster* and *Computer* from English and *Espresso* from Italian together with the items. English borrowed excessively from French after the Norman Conquest in 1066 when French was the language of the court. *Pork*, *mutton*, *veal* or *beef* were borrowed during that period and are nowadays completely integrated into the English language as can be seen in their spelling (Moessner 2003). Sometimes, sounds may be borrowed as well. An example of this is the /!/ sound represented orthographically by <x> in Xhosa (a Bantu language) that was borrowed from the neighbouring Khoisan languages (e.g. *uxolo* = 'excuse me'). Moreover, idioms or structures larger than one word may be borrowed. This can be seen in current German expressions such as *am Ende des Tages*= engl. 'at the end of the day', *nicht wirklich*= 'not really', *ich erinnere das*= 'I remember this' and the declining use of the definite article with the countries Iran and Iraq that used to have one in German.

Similar to the change of the borrowed material and its functions in the source language, material borrowed from spoken into sign languages is also changed formally and functionally. In terms of formal change, mouthings are no longer voiced as they would be as spoken language items and might become reduced as in TYPE 5 mouthings. Their function is obviously adapted to the visual-gestural modality.

Secondly, mouth gestures certainly seem to be sign language inherent and are only peripherally affected by language contact. This is shown by the fact that the frequency of mouth gestures – although not completely stable – does not change as dramatically as the other categories across age groups. Although a downward trend is visible in the data, I do not think that this kind of mouth action is ever going to disappear altogether, due to the importance of mouth gestures for the lexical and grammatical level of sign languages.

Thirdly and finally, the decrease in the category "no mouth action" entails an increase in the use of mouth actions in general. Thus, it can be inferred that younger signers use more mouth actions than older signers. Moreover, the great discrepancy between the general use of mouth actions in men and women in the oldest age group has almost been levelled in the youngest age groups. This also shows that signers nowadays tend to use more mouth actions than they used in older generations. This fact seems to be related to the increasing use of mouthings in both sexes and would thus ultimately be related to cross-modal language contact.

Before closing this chapter, I would like to address two alternative reasons for the developments of mouthings outlined in this section. They were first proposed in Mohr (2012).

The first proposal is that children might be copying their mothers which might lead to an increased use of English mouthings. In research on code-switching and code-blending in sign languages, the influence of the input to the children from their mothers on their output has been investigated (e.g. Baker & van den Bogaerde 2008). It has been shown that, although the input certainly does play a role for the output of the children (and later on, adults), it is not the only factor that influences the deaf children's language. In the NGT-Dutch study it was shown that deaf children produce less NGT/Dutch code-blended utterances than their mothers and a considerable amount of NGT. This shows that they emancipated themselves from the language use of their mothers which is also shown in the overall finding of the study, stating that three factors influence a child's language use: the child's ability in both languages, the input from the mothers and their own language choice. This language choice probably becomes more important as the children grow into adults which could then account for the results obtained in the current study on ISL. The fact that sign language is the natural language choice of Deaf communities despite its critical status at the level of traditional transmission (Plaza Pust 2005) emphasizes this fact. Moreover, this is also in line with the statistics. It is clearly visible that the use of mouthings increases (sometimes dramatically) from one generation to the next which could not be explained by a theory of simply copying the mothers. In that case, figures would have to stay the same for all age groups and they could not be different for men and women of the same age group. Men and women would be copying their mothers in the same way so this argument does not seem very plausible. Furthermore, the fact whether a mother or parent is deaf and uses sign language does not seem to play a role in this case either. Hence, signers from D/deaf families use the same amount of mouthings or even more than signers from hearing families. This is shown in table 5.3 below (the table is a modified version of Table 3 from Mohr 2012:196).

Table 5.3 Correlation of mouthings and language of family communication during childhood

	Language of communication at home[64]		
	ISL	English	Home sign
> 30% mouthings	0	1	1
30–70% mouthings	2	4	3
< 70% mouthings	1	1	2

As can be seen, there is no direct correlation between mouthings and the language of family communication during childhood. Thus, only one signer who uses more than 70% mouthings with his signs used English to communicate with his family, a figure that should have been higher if the copying hypothesis held true. Altogether, the argument that children might copy their mothers and thus use more mouthings seems not to be applicable to the ISL data.

The second proposal is that signers might be more bilingual now than they used to be several years ago. This argument cannot as easily be discarded with as the last one. Actually, this claim could be in line with the finding that language contact might be the reason for the increasing use of mouthings. The enforced language contact due to oralist education policies might indeed have caused a higher degree of ISL-English bilingualism in signers. In Mohr (2012) I also discuss the possibility that the concept of mono- and bilingualism has to be reformulated for sign languages as even in a potentially monolingual sign situation involving only native signers, both the signed and the spoken language seem to be "on" (Emmorey et al. 2005). This is emphasized by findings from Grosjean (2008) who mentions that signers rarely find themselves towards the monolingual end ("monolingual" being defined the traditional way) of the language mode continuum.

Moreover, studies on deaf communities and their developments and structures (Woll & Ladd 2003) mention that the socializing patterns of middle-aged and young deaf people in Western societies have changed radically during the past 30 years. There has been a general shift from deaf clubs, traditionally one of the two cornerstones of deaf communities[65] to more public settings which might ultimately lead to a change from an "oppositional community" to an "integrated" one.[66] This greater integration of young Deaf people into the hearing community might indeed lead to them having a more considerable knowledge of the ambient spoken language or showing an increased degree of bilingualism. However, I think that this is not the only reason for the developments shown in the statistics. A higher degree of bilingualism in signers seems not to be the first and foremost reason for the increasing use of mouthings but rather an accompanying language contact phenomenon. Consequently, the main reason for the developments outlined so far seems to be the different education policies at the Cabra schools.

As a conclusion to this chapter it can be stated that the hypotheses set up in section 4.1 were all proven by the analysis of the corpus data: the use of mouth actions in ISL is influenced by a signer's sex and women use more mouthings than men. Moreover, the use of mouth actions in ISL is influenced by a signer's age and older signers use less mouthings than younger ones. The considerable differences between individual signers hint at the fact that mouthings entered ISL as foreign language, borrowed material. These differences become smaller in younger generations so that it can be inferred that mouthings have become firmly integrated into ISL and that language change took place within the past 50–60 years.

These findings also confirm earlier claims that a) differences between male and female signing permeate the lexical level and extend to discourse or non-manual features (Leeson & Grehan 2004) and b) older signers use less mouthings than younger ones (Ó Baoill & Matthews 2000).

Chapter 6
Mouth Actions in ISL – Linguistic Factors

Having looked at the sociolinguistics of mouth actions in ISL in the previous chapter, the following elaborates on correlations between linguistic factors and mouth actions. Interrelations between mouth actions and word classes in sign languages have been recently mentioned in the literature (e.g. Crasborn et al. 2008; Schwager & Zeshan 2008; Meir 2012). They are claimed to be a modality-specific tool for PoS classifications in sign languages. More explicitly, these correlations are argued to hold between the morphological complexity of a sign and the different kinds of mouth actions. Morphologically more complex structures have been found to correlate with mouth gestures, in opposition to morphologically simple signs that were found to correlate with mouthings. The issue of morphological complexity needs further explanation here. While the immense morphological possibilities of verbs are often specifically mentioned in the literature and will be elaborated on later in this chapter, lexemes belonging to other word classes, such as nominal compounds, are admittedly morphologically complex as well. However, with respect to compounds I hypothesize that a) "dvandva" compounds typical of sign languages (Sandler & Lillo-Martin 2006; Meir 2012) need mouthings for meaning disambiguation and in order to compensate the semantic drift that occurred with the individual components. Dvandva compounds are constructions in which all parts are equal, i.e. no part modifies another. A typical example of this phenomenon is the ASL sign FRUIT composed of the (shortened) signs for BANANA/APPLE/CHERRY [etc.]. Morphological complexity will not be the driving force for mouth action occurrence in this case. Typical noun compounds found in spoken languages (noun + noun compounds, for instance), will be analyzed as well. Concerning this kind of sign, I further hypothesize b) that the mouthings of the individual nouns forming the compound will be maintained as they are closely linked to the individual items in endocentric compounds[67], whereas a new mouthing has to develop for exocentric compounds.

As was shown above, morphological complexity serves as the main criterion on which the broader hypotheses of this chapter are based. However, in special cases such as the ones mentioned above, other factors such as the semantics in relation to the form of the sign play an important role. The data from the SOI will be analyzed with respect to this point. This investigation on the one hand tries to verify the fact that a certain kind of mouth action frequently co-occurs with a certain word class and on the other hand tries to provide a first step towards an empirical analysis of word classes in the language. While a differentiation of word classes in ISL has been assumed by most researchers working on the language (e.g. Ó Baoill & Matthews 2000; Leeson 2001), this distinction has never been empirically investigated. Viewed the results of earlier studies on other sign languages, I expect morphologically complex signs or lexical classes like verbs (in case they exist in ISL), to occur most frequently with mouth gestures, while morphologically less complex signs or lexical classes like nouns will occur most frequently with mouthings.

Analyzing the data in reference to the hypotheses set up here, the chapter is structured as follows. The first part provides a theoretical background on word class research in spoken as compared to signed languages. In the second part of the chapter, the data from the SOI are analyzed in order to determine the syntactic categories and lexical classes of ISL. In the third and last part, correlations between mouth actions and the previously determined PoS of ISL will be tackled.

6.1. Word Classes – Historical and Theoretical Background

While all known languages seem to make some kind of distinction between major classes of words, word classes or parts-of-speech[68] vary immensely in quality and number between individual spoken languages (Schachter 1985). Questions of which distinctions are universal and which are language-specific play a crucial role, especially in typological linguistic research (Evans & Levinson 2010) while they are rather neglected in generative theory (Croft 2000). Linguistically distinct word classes have been acknowledged by scholars as far back as antiquity and are even considered to be "one of the most fundamental traits of human cognition" (Rijkhoff 2007; Evans & Levinson 2010; Rauh 2010) and one of the central elements of the linguistic analysis of a language (Erlenkamp 2000). However, the classification of linguistic elements into different classes is rather controversial. Rauh (2010) provides a very thorough account of the differences in word class distinctions in the framework of different linguistic theories. One of the central issues in theories on word class distinction is whether a categorization of words is functional or categorial (Sasse 1993b). Different opinions expressed with respect to this point reflect the theoretical framework of the respective researcher as supporting either a semantic, syntactic or morphosyntactic approach. Irrespective of the current theoretical standing of a certain researcher, all theories go back to the traditional word class categorization of ancient Greek.

The system of categorization of linguistic entities thus developed and used in Western grammatical theory, became one of the most integral parts of formal grammar. The development towards present-day linguistic theories of word class distinction can be divided into three periods (Sasse 1993b; Erlenkamp 2000). These will be outlined in the following.

The first period is the phase of the development and firm establishment of traditional word class distinction. It is also the longest of all three periods, extending from Plato's time until the 18th century. Plato as well as Aristotle utilized a mix of morphological, syntactic and semantic criteria for the distinction of word classes. While they only distinguished two different classes, later approaches extended the system to eight and acknowledged the complementary distribution of syntactic and morphological criteria in parts-of-speech distinction. Priscian was first to apply this system to another language, Latin. Although a development of the classification of parts-of-speech in this first period is certainly present, it completely lacked a theoretical discussion of this classification.

In the second period, starting in the 18th century, researchers started to criticize the traditional distinction of words, leading to the development of different approaches to word class distinction in the 1930s. They were primarily concerned with the question of whether word classes are morphological, syntactic or semantic classes and started to raise the issue of the choice of criteria for parts-of-speech distinction for the first time.

Finally, the third period which started with American structuralism, constitutes a break with traditional grammar and its distinction of word classes. Moreover, the question of the universality of word classes and their theoretical status, given a universal grammar, arose. According to the binary features applied in Universal Grammar, four main word classes could be distinguished: nouns, adjectives, verbs and prepositions.

Having outlined the history of word class distinction, its development from antiquity to present-day theories has been made clear. However, the traditional categorization of words established by the Ancient Greeks has never been completely abandoned (Sasse 1993b; Erlenkamp 2000). This is evident in the general discussion on the question of whether all categories are universal cross-linguistically. While it has been generally acknowledged that some word classes, like adjectives, are not found in all languages of the world, the general distinction between nouns and verbs is rather controversial. This distinction, which is very clear-cut in the Indo-European language family, is by no means universal when applied cross-linguistically. Eskimo, just as the Uralic and Altaic languages, is an often cited example of a language family that does not have verbs because they are actually nouns (Sasse 1993b). The opposite claim is often made for some American Indian languages such as the Salishan languages. Kinkade (1983) proposes a general distinction into full words and particles only. This distinction is based on the basic split of categories into full and function words that are often assumed in parts-of-speech research. Full words refer to items that have clear semantic content, while functional items usually arise by way of grammaticization and function as markers of syntactic functions (Sasse 1993b). Broschart (1987) agrees, claiming that nouns and verbs cannot be distinguished for these languages on formal grounds and are at best two sub-categories of a larger category of full words. The Philippine language Tagalog is very similar to the Salishan languages in that it also shows a distinction between full words and particles only (Himmelmann 1987; 2008). The languages of the Iroquoian family are also difficult concerning the general noun-verb distinction, however, they behave very differently from the language families mentioned so far. In Cayuga, e.g., all full words are inflected for person and hence are all predicative – the language was even considered by Sasse (1993b) not to have any nouns at all. However, other researchers such as Mithun (2000) convincingly state that the Iroquoian languages do indeed have a noun category.

It can thus be stated that although a universal noun-verb distinction was taken for granted by many researchers for a long time, it is not ubiquitous in the languages of the world. Rather, there is a continuum ranging from clear-cut distinctions to theoretical non-distinction of nouns and verbs (Sasse 1993b). This continuum is arranged around the prototypes of nouns and verbs, relating to the fact of gradience of word classes, thus entailing prototypical and less prototypical members of the respective classes. The prototype approach to word classes is described in detail in section 6.1.1.

Diachronically, languages might move within this continuum Sasse (Sasse 1993b:660 f.). It is hence noteworthy that the number of parts-of-speech categories of individual languages might change drastically over time as historical developments might not only affect the noun and verb classes but all lexical categories of a language.

Contrary to the noun-verb distinction, the closed class of pro-forms is a class that seems universal cross-linguistically (Sasse 1993b:669). More traditionally, these items are called "pronouns", however, it seems noteworthy that Sasse (1993b) uses the broader term "pro-forms" to acknowledge the possibility of pro-verbs, pro-sentences, etc. and the fact that these forms are usually not a single class. Traditionally, grammarians divided the class into personal, reflexive, reciprocal, possessive, demonstrative, relative, interrogative and indefinite pronouns. This distinction, as it is based on classical Latin, is rather euro-centric, however, and does not acknowledge the reality of other non-Indo-European languages that do not have as many sub-classifications. The most central class, namely personal pronouns, is elaborated on below.

Functionally, this word class is defined as substituting a member of the corresponding full-word category, as shifting reference and as having deictic function (Greenberg 1986; Sasse 1993b; Evans 2000). Supporting the fact that they are central to the pronoun class is the fact that the occurrence of personal pronouns in the world's languages is nearly universal. However, a sub-categorization of the class proves rather controversial. While it is generally acknowledged that the class is organized along person and number lines (Evans 2000; Helmbrecht 2004), the feature person itself is problematic. Sasse (1993b:670) states that three persons are found universally, namely first person (that of the speaker), second person (that of the addressee) and third person (that of an entity that is neither speaker nor addressee) while Greenberg (1986:XIIX) claims that first and second person are more central to the class, as many languages do not have a third person pronoun that is distinct from one or more demonstratives (Greenberg 1986; Sasse 1993b; Helmbrecht 2004). Helmbrecht (2004) elaborates on the reason for this controversy: he states that there is a major functional division between first and second person pronouns as shifters (of refence) on the one hand and third person pronouns relating anaphoric and cataphoric reference on the other.[69]

The outline of the controversy around a universal noun-verb distinction in the languages of the world and the description of personal pronouns has shown that different researchers indeed apply different parameters to parts-of-speech distinctions. For the noun-verb distinction, for instance, the notions gradience, centre of a category and prototype were mentioned. These are taken from semantic approaches to word class distinctions. Apart from these semantic accounts, there are also syntactic and morphosyntactic theories of parts-of-speech categorizations. Along with an outline of the different theories on word classes in sign languages, these different approaches will be discussed in the following sections.

6.1.1. Semantic Approaches to Word Class Distinction

Although it has been pointed out in the literature that a purely semantic categorization of words is impossible (e.g. Schachter 1985; Sasse 1993b), some textbooks divide words into classes according to semantic criteria. This is also called the "notional approach" (e.g. Croft 2000). A purely semantic account of word class categorization is Jackendoff (1983). Hence, nouns are claimed to denote persons or things, verbs to refer to actions, processes and states and adjectives to properties (Dixon 1982; Sasse 1993b). They occupy an intermediate position between nouns, which usually express completely time-stable things or concepts, and verbs, which mostly refer to rapidly changing states of affairs. Although this kind of distinction is very intuitive, it fails to account for the enormous amount of disagreement between lexical and semantic classes in many languages. Abstract nouns, for instance, present obvious problems. Thus, nouns denoting concepts like ‘ugliness’ or ‘jealousy’ are difficult to classify as “things” while they still have nominal character and are thus classified as nouns in languages such as English or German. Moreover, the existence of synonyms mapped onto different word classes in different languages is problematic for a purely semantic account. Evans (2000) cites the French verbs *savoir* and *ignorer* and their English counterparts *know* and *be ignorant of* as a case in point. Conversion, as in English words like *kiss* (verb) and *kiss* (noun), is another argument that proves the deficiency of purely semantic approaches to parts-of-speech categorization.

However, Sasse (1993b) emphasizes that the semantic criterion cannot be discarded altogether. Consequently, he proposes to consider a semantic viewpoint for a general motivation of universal word class distinction, which might serve as a point of departure for language-specific morphosyntactic analyses of word classes. The classification of human impressions of the real world into various semantic groups such as materials, states, processes, etc. could be utilized for a rough universal categorization into different lexical and semantic classes (Sasse 1993b:648).

Another semantic analysis is put forth by researchers postulating a prototype approach to parts-of-speech categorization. In her theory of semantic primitives, Wierzbicka (2000) claims there are universal semantic exemplars of every part-of-speech category that are based on a set of universally lexicalized concepts that emerged from empirical cross-linguistic investigation carried out in the “Natural Semantic Metalanguage” framework (cf. e.g. Wierzbicka 1996). In the noun category, PERSON and THING are universal lexical primitives of nouns. For verbs, DO and HAPPEN are universal lexical exemplars. The universal semantic exemplars of the adjectival category are BIG and SMALL. She further mentions I and YOU as universal semantic exemplars of the pronoun category. In a second step, she combines her theory with universal syntax. According to her, universal semantic exemplars are to be preferred over a general notional account because they are more concrete than the broad generalizations put forth by for example Schachter and Sasse and at the same time more general than

Dixon's "semantic type" approach, since they are based on universal conceptual primitives (Wierzbicka 2000:289).

Another key term in the context of semantic approaches, especially prototype theories, is gradience. Publications such as Croft (1991), Knobloch & Schaeder (2000) and Evans (2000) have mentioned the issue of (semantic) gradience of word class membership for language specific as well as universal parts-of-speech categorization. The theory of gradience in word class membership is based on prototype theory stating that there are always core (prototypical) members of a certain category and other members that are at the periphery of the category in question. The core members therefore display all of the semantic characteristics of the category, while the peripheral members show only some of them and lack others. Croft (1991) thus states that prototypical nouns refer to objects, have zero valency and refer to stative, persistent and non-gradable entities. Concrete nouns are hence prototypical category members, while a more abstract noun like *change* lacks the characteristic of stativity and is consequently a more peripheral member of the category. It is also noteworthy that these non-prototypical members of a class are most likely to show cross-linguistic variation in parts-of-speech membership. While prototype approaches to word class categorization are generally very much favoured in current word class theories, some researchers such as Erlenkamp (2000) question the applicability of prototype theory to the problem of parts-of-speech distinction (especially with reference to sign language). She refers to the fact that prototype theory is originally a theory from the domain of cognitive psychology and cannot easily be applied to other subject matters such as linguistics and word class distinction.

While it is undeniable that prototype theory did not originate in the domain of linguistics, I do not see its application to word class distinction as problematic as Erlenkamp. Her central criticism seems to be that the establishment of prototypical and less prototypical members of a word class is totally arbitrary and not verifiable by any metalinguistic means. However, if prototype theory is applied to linguistics, it is only reasonable to apply linguistic (instead of metalinguistic) criteria to the establishment of categories. Although these are not easily identifiable and applicable cross-linguistically, they are more or less unproblematic when looking at single languages as they are determined culturally. Therefore, I suggest that prototype theory seems rather plausible in the context of parts-of-speech classification and should not be summarily discarded. I also agree with the aforementioned authors in that there certainly are prototypical and rather peripheral members of categories and that this fact accounts for a lot of the linguistic diversity that can be observed around the world.[70] However, we should keep in mind that most category definitions are rather euro-centric, resulting in the Indo-European word classes being at the centre of every category, while less studied languages' parts-of-speech are almost always at the periphery.[71]

Especially interesting in this respect are what we call adjectival concepts in Indo-European languages. To date, it remains unclear why some languages show a distinct adjective class while others do not. Rijkhoff (2000), for instance, follows up on the claim that adjectives only occur in languages in which the numeral is in a direct construction with a noun (but not vice versa). He finds out that this is only partly true, as the occurrence of adjectives seems to be linked to a certain lexical feature that is typically absent in classifier languages. Hence, in languages which use nouns with the semantic feature [-Shape], there is no way of distinguishing between nouns and adjectives, resulting in the languages apparently not having a distinct adjective class.

However, languages without an adjective class or with a relatively small and closed class, employ other strategies in order to express property concepts. Dixon (1982) investigates adjectival concepts in seventeen different languages, analyzing how languages with a small closed adjective class express the concepts that are referred to by adjectives in adjectival languages. For his theory, Dixon postulates a semantic account and relies on prototype theory (Dixon 1982:12).[72]

Typologically, there are two kinds of languages: those that have an open adjective class by which all seven semantic types are expressed, and languages that have a closed adjective class in which only some of the seven universal semantic types are present. Moreover, the notion of gradience can also be applied to the adjective class: languages can be situated along a continuum from strongly adjectival languages (in which all seven universal types are associated with the adjective class), to strongly verbal ones (in which the marked pole of an adjectival opposition is usually expressed by a verb while the unmarked one is represented by an adjective or noun) to neutral (in which for some oppositions the marked pole is realized as a verb but where the majority of cases is associated with only one single part-of-speech).

While the above facts do not repudiate prototype theory, they certainly question our traditional parts-of-speech classifications. Sasse's statement that although a purely semantic approach does not suffice to distinguish word classes on a universal level, the semantic criterion should not be discarded with and be taken into account for parts-of-speech classifications, is surely the most important issue to be kept in mind in this respect.

6.1.2. Syntactic Approaches to Word Class Distinction

The syntactic level is central for parts-of-speech distinctions, especially to generativist accounts of word class categorizations. This is reflected by terminology: many researchers refer to word classes as "syntactic categories".[73] A categorization of words according to syntactic criteria reflects the view that word classes are functional rather than categorial in nature (Sasse 1993b). Whether this claim can actually bear up against critical analysis will be discussed in the following paragraphs.

Applying the syntactic criterion, researchers like Benveniste (1966) mention that ultimately, word class distinctions are subsidiary to syntax and certain syntactic slots like subject or predicate. Consequently, nouns are predisposed to be subjects and usually function as arguments, verbs are predisposed to be predicates and typically head a clause, while adjectives may function either as dependents of nouns or as predicates (Evans 2000). However, this view faces similar problems as a purely semantic approach. It lacks absoluteness as nouns do not always coincide with the subject of a clause just as verbs do not always fill the predicate slot. Hengeveld et al. (2004) divide languages into those that have a rigid parts-of-speech system and those that have a flexible one. Flexible systems have only one class to fill all syntactic slots (like Samoan, for example[74]), while rigid ones have extremely specialized classes (Tuscarora for instance). In flexible languages that have only one class, this class of words fills both syntactic slots, i.e. no predisposition for any syntactic constituent can be observed. Therefore, the claim that word classes are purely functional in nature does not seem plausible. Further, these facts hint at the insufficiency of the syntactic criterion alone for a parts-of-speech distinction.

Besides Hengeveld (1992, 2004), there are other syntactic approaches to word class distinctions in the world's languages. Croft (2000) especially emphasizes distributional (syntactic) analysis as a major tool in parts-of-speech categorization because it provides the complete picture of the grammatical patterning of a language and might reveal covert categories. However, it might also uncover fuzzy category behaviour at the boundaries of the established classes. This relates to the aforementioned prototype analysis of categories and gradience theory, which Croft clearly supports, stating that category membership is not always clear-cut for individual lexical items. What is more, Croft himself admits to certain flaws of the distributional analysis approach. Consequently, he states that distributional analysis alone cannot determine whether in some cases a separate class analysis or a subclass analysis should be preferred.

Another criterion that can be directly linked to the syntactic analysis of word classes is the pragmatic or discourse criterion. Since sentence structure is often dependent on the larger discourse that sentences are embedded in, researchers have attempted to derive the basic noun-verb distinction from discourse categories such as topic and comment (Hopper & Thompson 1984; 1985). Especially Hopper and Thompson (1985) have emphasized the fact that the topic function seems to coincide with the category of nouns cross-linguistically, while the comment function is usually reserved for verbs. They hypothesize that the nature of nouns originates in the need for a word class that functions as introductory of participants and props, whereas verbs are ideally made up to report events.

As has become apparent, a purely syntactic or discourse account for word class categorization is equally insufficient as a purely semantic one. However, I agree with Sasse (1993b) that, just as the semantic criterion, a syntactic discourse based account might help in understanding the general mechanisms of word class categorization.

6.1.3. Morphosyntactic Approaches to Word Class Distinction

The morphosyntactic criterion is central to the distinction of form classes in the Classical languages that were ultimately defined by their inflexional composition. Hence, the observation that lexical categories behave differently with respect to their ability to take inflections and thus create different forms, was crucial for parts-of-speech categorization (Sasse 1993b). The main distinction between category-establishing and category-changing morphology was also made relatively early. While the first indicates the general functions of a category, as tense, aspect, mood and person do for verbs, the latter is concerned with deferring lexemes from one category to another (by means of derivational morphology, for example). Both kinds of morphology can be used to define the characteristics of word classes in a single language. Nevertheless, it is not valid for a cross-linguistic account of word classes and is therefore not universal.

Firstly, the morphosyntactic account is not without flaws because the notions of gradience and prototype play important roles just as in semantic theories. In those languages that show morphological inflections for nouns, they typically inflect for number, gender and case. Consequently, these grammatical categories are at the centre of the prototypical morphological criteria defining nouns. Evans (2000) mentions that number and gender inflections usually reflect characteristics of the referent while case inflections provide information on the syntactic function of the noun in the clause. He cites Russian as an example of an Indo-European language in which nouns are inflected for all three and also govern adjectival agreement concerning these features. Less prototypical morphological information represented on the noun are the aforementioned inflections for tense or mood in some languages of the Tupí-Guaraní family. A final grammatical category that is relatively widespread among the languages of Africa, the Caucasus and Australia is that of nominal class. Class systems categorize nouns into subsets, usually on a semantic basis. The class systems found in many African languages, however, are highly grammaticized and their semantic basis is hence no longer clearly visible (Sasse 1993b). Gender systems found in many Indo-European languages are often considered to be equal to the noun class systems found in non-Indo-European languages (Aikhenvald 2000; Grinevald 2000). However, they show a more limited semantic motivation of assignment to classes and are often portmanteau morphemes combining other grammatical categories such as number and case.[75]

Turning to the category of verbs, cross-linguistically, they are the word class with the most complex morphological possibilities (especially in polysynthetic languages like Nahuatl, for example). Evans (2000:712) lists tense, aspect, mood, negation, voice, reflexives, reciprocals, applicatives, person, number, gender, object-definiteness, markers of switch-reference, logophoricity, honorifics or conjugation membership as the most common ones. Moreover, there are numerous possibilities to morphologically derive other lexical classes from verbs, as for instance nominalizers or participal morphology transforming verbs into modifiers. Prototypically, verbs inflect for tense, aspect, mood and person. There are however languages in which other categories show one of the aforementioned inflections. In Hausa, for example, what seem to be pronouns when applying syntactic and semantic criteria, inflect for tense and mood, a rather exceptional historical development that Hayward (2000) has commented on.

Not only is the verb class able to show the most complex morphological phenomena, but it can also be further subdivided into smaller sub-classes according to different criteria. Looking at argument structure, the subclasses of intransitive, transitive, ditransitive, semi-transitive or subjectless can be established (Evans 2000). Two other sub-classes that are often observed are copula and auxiliaries. However, it is noteworthy that while some languages consider the first as a sub-class of verbs, other languages have a special class of copulas, like Hausa, for instance. The latter verbal sub-class, namely auxiliaries, usually "form a closed class of words encoding information about inflectional categories typically morphologically associated with verbs and with the clause level in terms of their scope" (Evans 2000:718). This class is far from universal though, as there are many languages that lack this category.

Finally, there are various languages with morphologically quite limited or closed verb classes. In these languages, predicate constructions are usually expressed by verb + preverb combinations. Evans (2000) lists Hindi and the Papuan languages Kalam and Kobon as examples of this kind of language. Additionally, these languages might employ the strategy of verb chaining in order to form complex predicate constructions.

Looking at adjectives, they prove to be a very heterogeneous class with respect to its morphological markers (cf. e.g. Dixon 1982; Croft 2000; Rijkhoff 2000). However, it can generally be stated that they usually do not take tense, aspect or mood inflections or specify for person and number.

Finally, a short comment on the closed class of pronouns seems noteworthy. Morphologically, they might show traits that are special for these forms. Hence, in Indo-European, many pronouns possess special case endings with no direct affinity to the noun. These kinds of discrepancies can also be found outside Indo-European, as in present day Arabic, for instance (Sasse 1993b).

Generalizing the morphological potential of the individual word classes compared to the abovementioned concrete examples, Croft's structural coding and behavioural potential criteria from his radical construction grammar framework add to the problem of the morphosyntactic criterion and prototype theory. According to his criteria, the marked (and thus less prototypical) member of a category is encoded by at least as many morphemes as the unmarked member.

Another flaw of the morphosyntactic account is isolating languages which rather employ word order and/or adpositions in order to convey categories like tense, mood, etc. Word classes in these languages have to be defined using either syntactic, semantic or a mix of both criteria since classes simply cannot be established on a morphosyntactic level. Furthermore, Evans (2000:711) mentions that many head-marking languages utilize pronominal agreement on the verb (and leaving the noun unmarked) in order to provide information about syntactic relations. Hence it becomes apparent that while morphosyntactic criteria are certainly among the most traditional and also for some languages the most clear-cut and convincing parameters for word class distinction, they are not sufficient on their own.

Sasse (1993b) proposes a morphosyntactic account for categorization as the starting point for parts-of-speech classification in one language, leading on to a syntactic and finally a semantic, universally applicable, account.[76]

Agreeing on that point, one criterion, be it semantic, syntactic-discourse related or morphosyntactic, does not suffice to account for a cross-linguistic distinction of word classes. While one linguistic level may certainly suffice for a parts-of-speech categorization in a single language, it cannot be applied cross-linguistically. Even the semantic criterion that seems to be closest to a universal criterion for word class distinction, fails to account for all languages. Its application as sole criterion for categorization would reflect the abovementioned euro-centric view of lexical classes that is certainly not appropriate for a typological analysis of word classes. It would completely fail to account for the diversity discovered in the systems of the world's languages (Haspelmath 2010).

6.1.4. Word Class Distinction in Sign Languages

While the distinction of word classes or parts-of-speech reaches back to antiquity for spoken language research and is an essential part of formal grammar, it remains an under-represented and neglected topic in sign linguistics (Schwager & Zeshan 2008; Meir 2012). There are several reasons for this neglect. Meir (2012:85) mentions three central issues that often complicate word class research in sign linguistics. Firstly, sign languages are articulated in another modality than spoken languages which makes word class distinctions hardly comparable to traditional classifications. Secondly, sign languages are much younger than most spoken languages, which is why they show different linguistic traits in general. Finally, the field of sign linguistics is rather young as compared to spoken language linguistics. The body of literature and research that sign linguists can draw upon is simply much smaller than that of spoken language linguistics.

The main issues concerning word class distinction in sign languages are related to the criteria used for establishing distinct categories. Firstly, there is an overlap between formational and meaningful functions of the sub-lexical parts of a sign. This results in the fact that phonemic features and morphemes cannot easily be distinguished from one another. Zeshan (2002:170) and Schwager and Zeshan (2008) also mention that the concept of duality of patterning is seriously challenged by sub-lexical parts of iconic signs which they claim to be meaningful on a sub-lexical level. For instance, the handshape feature of a sign might be exploited for its iconic potential and become meaningful within the discourse (a special case of phonosymbolism (Stokoe 1960; Mandel 1980)). Currently, there is no widely accepted overt definition of the morpheme unit in sign languages (Schwager & Zeshan

2008). Moreover, the notion of 'word' is equally problematic with respect to sign languages. While many researchers claim that most signs are monomorphemic (Zeshan 2002; Zwitserlood 2003; Schwager & Zeshan 2008; Meir 2012), and the concepts of grammatical and phonological word can be applied meaningfully to sign languages although the first is weakened due to non-concatenative morphology, there are signs that elude the definition of a monomorphemic sign. However, it is generally accepted that the definition of a phonological word adheres to the following constraints (Sandler 1999): it is monosyllabic, it uses only one set of fingers for its handshape, it uses only one major body area and it obeys constraints on two-handed combinations. Besides, Zeshan categorizes signs into three types according to morphological and semantic criteria, namely phonosymbols, arbitrary signs and classifiers.

While some researchers consider the abovementioned critical cases to be indeed morphologically complex signs (Zwitserlood 2003), others have come up with special terms in order to avoid the notion of morphological complexity in this respect. The issue of compounds also remains fairly unresolved as far as sign language morphology is concerned.[77]

As was outlined above, the morphological criterion is problematic as far as word class distinction in sign languages is concerned. Due to their rather young age, sign languages have not had the chance to develop a large amount of inflectional morphology (Meir 2012). Adding to the aforementioned facts is the problem of morphological marking that, when it occurs, often cannot be related to word class establishment (Schwager & Zeshan 2008). Only very few word class determining affixes are mentioned for sign languages. Aronoff et al. (2005) report a class of prefix deriving verbs in IsSL. These prefixes consist of pointing to a sense organ, the mouth or head and conveying the meaning of 'to X by (eye)/hearing (ear) thinking/ (head)/intuiting (nose)/ saying (mouth)'. A suffix attaching to nouns and adjectives in IsSL and forming adjectives is mentioned in Meir (2004), Meir and Sandler (2008) and Meir (2012). It can be glossed as -NOT-EXIST and is equivalent to the English suffix *–less*. Meir et al. (2010) comment on toponymic compounds in ABSL which usually consist of a pointing sign in the second part of the construction.

Besides problematic issues related to morphology, the syntactic behaviour of sign languages has not been sufficiently researched to be a reliable criterion for word class assignment. Despite the fact that the body of research on ASL syntax is relatively large, little is known about the syntax of other, smaller sign languages. Padden (1988) tried to establish three major open word classes and three verbal subclasses for ASL based on syntactic grounds.

Hence, she argued that ASL nouns can be modified by quantifiers, adjectives can be inflected for intensive aspect while verbs are defined negatively in that they cannot be combined with quantifiers and cannot be pre-modifiers of other signs. The tests Padden used for her study prove problematic for other sign languages and her results are thus not universally applicable. This situation is therefore similar to morphosyntactic criteria for word class distinction in spoken languages as these cannot be applied cross-linguistically as well.

A traditional notional analysis of parts-of-speech for sign languages has been attempted as well. Schwager and Zeshan (2008:520, ff.) put forth a feature analysis of DGS and Kata Kolok. They assume eight semantic classes (person/thing, event, property, place, time, relation, quantity and situation, based on Stassen (1997) and Anward (2000)) and a subdivision into subclasses based on the ontological classification of Aristotle and Dionysius Thrax. Relying on semantic feature analysis, they deny the idea of gradience of category membership and prototype theory. This seems rather problematic, looking at the discussion of this approach in the previous sections of this chapter. Based on the previous semantic classification, they map the individual classes on syntactic roles and morphological operations. Altogether, their analysis presents a comprehensive account of word class distinctions in sign languages and illustratively depicts cross-linguistic differences in parts-of-speech classifications in sign languages.

Finally, Zeshan (2000) suggests a modality-specific classification of word classes in IPSL. Signs are thus classified according to spatial characteristics, i.e. signs that cannot move in space at all, signs produced in neutral space, etc. Even though this account is certainly innovative and maybe even accurate for the language discussed, it has been criticized for its inapplicability to larger cross-linguistic comparisons with spoken languages (Meir 2012).

After these fairly general remarks on problematic issues arising in the distinction of word classes in sign languages, I will briefly comment on concrete problems concerning those word classes that are undisputed among sign linguists. These are almost all open classes, namely nouns, verbs and adjectives. Moreover, pronominal systems in sign languages will be discussed as they are essential for verb morphology in sign languages, which is highly relevant for correlations with mouth actions.

An issue that has brought forth a considerable amount of research and literature is the distinction of similar or even phonologically identical noun-verb pairs in the sign languages of the world. Pairs like these have been described for ASL (Lillo-Martin 2005), LIS (Pizzuto & Corazza 1996), Auslan (Johnston 2001) and for Langue des Signes Québécoise (LSQ) (Bouchard et al. 2005; Voghel 2005) to name but a few. Generally, there is said to be a derivational relationship between nouns and verbs. An important criterion in this respect is the different movement patterns of the two sign classes: verbs show single, unrestrained, long movement while nouns display repeated, restrained, short movement. This can be related to the fact that in verbs, repetition of movement may convey what has been called aspect in the literature, such as iterative or durative (Voghel 2005). However, Johnston (2001) mentions that with respect to his studies on Auslan, repetition alone does not seem to be a productive nominal derivational process, although it is generally true that 57% of the nouns in their data showed repeated movement (1.5 movement cycles) while 79% of the verbs showed only single movement. It might be possible that this process is only productive in certain sign languages while it is not in others.

Moreover, some researchers mention the different possibilities of morphological marking on verbs and nouns. Hence, verbs can be marked for tense, person[78], number and take negation; predicates can be marked for aspect. However, according to Padden's (1988) tripartite verb class distinction, not all verbs participate in this agreement system. Also, it is claimed that neither nouns nor verbs can be marked for gender in ASL. This, too, may hint at cross-linguistic variation concerning this feature. Furthermore, nouns can be used with the possessive while verbs cannot. They are also assigned a spatial locus while most verbs only reuse spatial loci. Moreover, adjectives are mentioned to function as verbs sometimes (Lillo-Martin 2005). My own interpretation of these items in ISL is discussed in 6.2.2.

What is more, almost all researchers working on the topic of noun-verb distinctions of meaning related, formally similar noun-verb pairs mention mouth actions as an important distinguishing feature. This holds true for all sign languages mentioned above (except Lillo-Martin (2005) on ASL). Johnston (2001) mentions that the mouthing of English words is more frequent with nouns while it only occurs with verbs in a minority of cases and might be a primary way to distinguish nouns from verbs in Auslan. He even claims it to be more significant than the oft-cited movement patterns. Voghel (2005) also mentions that word mouthings usually accompany nouns in LSQ while "expressive mouth movements" (= mouth gestures) occur more frequently with verbs. She concludes that word mouthing and expressive mouth movements seem intimately linked to a certain category. The validity of this claim with respect to ISL will be investigated in section 6.2.

Finally, a completely different view of the problematic issues related to a noun-verb distinction in sign languages shall be mentioned. In her work on syntactic categories and lexical classes in German Sign Language, Erlenkamp (2000) claims that a noun category does not exist in DGS. According to her analysis, there are only two syntactic categories in DGS, namely verbs and multifunctional signs, and five lexical classes.[79] Meir (2012) also mentions the abundance of multifunctional signs in the world's sign languages. Erlenkamp's approach is certainly an interesting theory that might be considered for other studies as well.

Before closing this section, a few comments on pronominal systems seem noteworthy. As in spoken languages, pronouns form a closed word class in sign languages. Major issues concerning pronouns in sign languages are firstly the similarity of definite determiners and pronouns, the motivatedness of pronouns as well as the controversy of which person distinctions can be made.

With respect to the first issue, it can be observed that pronouns and definite determiners may be identical in phonological form. Hence, pointers (indeces)[80] can function either as pronouns or as definite determiners, depending on the context (Lillo-Martin 2005). In case the pointer initially assigns a locus, it functions as a determiner, if it refers back to a specific referent, it is a pronoun. This shows that phonological or morphological criteria alone do not suffice in order to determine a sign's category but that their use in the larger discourse is essential.

Concerning the motivatedness of pronominal systems in sign languages, indexicality is the key feature to be mentioned. Therefore, all indexic signs, pronouns being one class, point to a location in space associated with a referent. This makes them seem very iconically motivated[81], and indeed Cormier (2007) mentions indexicality as one type of visual motivation. However, pronominal reference in sign languages is linguistic in terms of morphology or discourse structure and not exclusively iconic. Moreover, pronouns are lexicalized with respect to their location. Nevertheless, there are some cases of non-indexic pronouns attested for ASL and BSL. Cormier (2007) found that not all pronouns point to their referents in the same way as plural pronouns in general are less indexic than singulars and first person plurals are more indexic than general plurals. She also found that this lack of indexicality in some pronouns is due to ease of articulation and general motor skills of the human body. Thus, signers might sometimes produce a pronoun at a location that is motorically easier, as ease of articulation may override indexicality. From a more theoretical point of view, Keller (1998) claims that the traditional spoken language distinction between deictic and anaphoric pronouns does not hold for sign languages and should be expanded by a generic term "chorophoric" (Keller 1998:66).

Finally, person distinctions in sign languages have been and still are rather controversial. While the first person is undisputed for all sign languages, it is not clear whether a further distinction between second and third person can be made as well or if the basic distinction is between first and non-first person only. Those that claim a three-person system are for example Friedman (1975) or Klima and Bellugi (1979). They postulate a system that distinguishes a first person (signer), a second person (addressee) and a third person (non-addressed third participants). This older view was replaced by a newer theory that does not refer to person in the context of pronouns at all, but to locations. The problem with the theory of the tripartite system is that each non-signer and non-addressed participant in a discourse would have the same value, namely third person (Cormier 2007). Moreover, there are theoretically an infinite number of third person values as far as locations in the signing space are concerned. Hence, many researchers nowadays argue in favour of a locus analysis, analyzing the loci as retrieving their content from the discourse (cf. e.g. Lacy 1974; Cormier et al. 1999; Cormier 2007). A third analysis of the pronoun system of sign languages claims a dual distinction into first and non-first person. This theory takes into account the special status that is assigned to the first person in sign languages across the world. According to Meier (1990) for instance, there is no grammatical distinction between a possible second or third person since the only distinction between reference to the addressee or a non-addressed third person is eye gaze (which is also not always a reliable criterion). This view is currently followed by many researchers, such as Lillo-Martin (1995), Emmorey (2002), Rathmann and Mathur (2002) or Zwitserlood (2003).

6.1.5. Discussion

Having outlined the different theories of word class research in spoken and signed languages, the present section provides a short summary and comparison of these theoretical bases.

The main difference between spoken and sign language word class research is that the first is an ancient discipline reaching as far back as antiquity, whereas the latter represents a relatively young field (just like all other sign linguistic research). While spoken language parts-of-speech analysis constitutes a major part of formal grammar, it is a fairly neglected topic in sign linguistic typological research. The most important reason for this is the relative youth of the discipline of sign linguistics in general. It is therefore not surprising that the mere lack of research on sign languages and their structures conditions many of the central problems concerning the distinction of categories. The inability to determine the border between phonological and morphological structures and the small number of studies on sign language syntax (other than that of ASL) are thus highly problematic. A purely notional, i.e. semantic, account of the distinction of word classes in sign languages would be as inadequate as it is for word classes in spoken languages. The problems with this framework were outlined in detail in section 6.1.1. Consequently, this fact represents one of the similarities between parts-of-speech categorization in spoken and signed languages.

Another similarity is the insufficiency of the application of one linguistic level as the basis for word class categorizations. As was shown, morphological and morphosyntactic, syntactic, discourse analytic and semantic accounts have to be combined in order to formulate cross-linguistically applicable theories. This holds true for languages from both modalities. However, sign languages, being from the visual gestural modality, have the advantage of being able to take other linguistic "levels", namely non-manual features and spatial relations, into account. This tool is therefore unavailable in spoken language research.

Finally, the theoretical basis for the empirical study in the next sections shall be outlined. As this book is primarily concerned with mouth actions, the importance of mouth actions for PoS classifications in ISL will be the main issue treated in the following section. However, I do not suggest that mouth actions are the only tool for a thorough analysis of parts-of-speech in ISL or any other sign language for that matter. In order to achieve a correct and typologically valid word class categorization, other linguistic levels have to be taken into account. Thus, I will follow for example Sasse's (1993) approach and utilize a combination of all abovementioned criteria for the analysis. The main criteria for syntactic categories and lexical classes that are going to be distinguished will be outlined in 6.2.

6.2. Mouth Actions and Word Classes in ISL

After having outlined the theoretical background of word class differentiation in spoken and signed languages, the second part of this chapter is concerned with the presentation and evaluation of the data from the Signs of Ireland Corpus. This analysis is essential for the later analysis of correlations between mouth actions and word classes as a thorough analysis of PoS distinctions in ISL is the prerequisite for a valid analysis of mouth action-PoS correlations. The current investigation is the first to empirically research word class distinctions in ISL. Other publications have simply presupposed the word classes of spoken English (e.g. nouns, verbs) but this analysis will investigate word class difference in ISL on the basis of typological theories of PoS distinctions. In line with other researchers such as Sasse (1993a, b), Erlenkamp (2000) and Rauh (2010), a difference between syntactic categories and lexical classes is made. Syntactic categories are therefore categories of formal characteristics that are related to the argument, predicate, etc. phrase while lexical classes are classes whose members display a certain composition of inherent characteristics that are distinct from the characteristics of other classes (Erlenkamp 2000:27). Sasse (1993a) mentions the importance of the disentanglement of the parameters applied for the establishment of word classes. He distinguishes four levels of parameterization (Sasse 1993a:196):[82]

1. **The formal parameter**: including inflection, derivation and distribution.
2. **The syntactic parameter**: slot-filler-relation, the mapping onto syntactic categories.
3. **The ontological-semantic parameter**: the mapping onto ontological categories and classes of meaning.
4. **The discourse-pragmatic parameter**: the mapping onto basic discourse functions (reference, predication, modification).

For most European languages, syntactic categories and lexical classes can be established and are identical. Sasse (1993a) calls these TYPE A languages. However, cross-linguistically, this is not always the case. Sasse mentions three other types of languages that can be found with respect to word classes. TYPE B languages have distinct syntactic categories and lexical classes which do, however, not correlate. An example of this is Tagalog or (according to Erlenkamp's analysis) DGS. TYPE C languages show distinct lexical classes but do not distinguish syntactic categories. Sasse's analysis of Cayuga provides an example of this kind of language. Finally, TYPE D languages only show distinct syntactic categories but do not differentiate lexical classes. Tongan is mentioned as an example of this kind of language (Sasse 1993a:200).

For ISL it remains to be shown which type of language it constitutes. Answering this question will be one of the central issues of this chapter. In order to do so, the four parameters mentioned above will be applied to ISL. With respect to the formal parameter, the supposed lexical class of nouns should be able to inflect for number and the possessive, while verbs can be marked for person, object, manner and aspect. Whether this can be proven with respect to the data will be part of the analysis. For the syntactic parameter, basic clause structure plays a crucial role. This has been found to be rather flexible. Leeson (2001) investigated basic clause structure as part of her study on verbal valency in ISL and found a general order theme-verb-undergoer for transitive sentences with plain verbs and theme-verb(-undergoer) for transitive sentences with morphologically marked verbs. The important thing to note here is that plain verbs usually pattern with overt arguments, while morphologically marked verbs pattern with implicit arguments as those are referred to by the referential loci of the verb. Moreover, classifier constructions (predicates) always have to be preceded by a referring NP.

While the above paragraph only outlines the formal and syntactic parameters for word class identification in general, a more detailed account will be provided in the following sections. The most important characteristic to be considered here is whether mouth actions can serve as a modality-specific tool for word class recognition in ISL. Finally, the issue of mouth gestures as a separate word class will be tackled. Due to their often reported and observed iconicity, they resemble ideophones in spoken languages as is discussed in section 6.2.4.

6.2.1. Syntactic Categories of ISL

Concerning the syntactic categories of ISL, I have looked exclusively at content words (signs) that would be able to fulfill the functions of predicate, argument or modifier. Predicates constitute the proposition of a sentence, arguments the theme of this proposition and modifiers may either modify the predicate (adverbial modifiers) or the argument (attributive modifiers). A few problematic issues concerning this point are the abovementioned free word order and the lack of a lexical copula to distinguish predicating, specifying and identifying predicates. Predicate and argument (S) are juxtaposed just as argument and attributive modifier. As there are usually no morphosyntactic markers for predicative or attributive use, it is inherently difficult to distinguish between the two. Examples of this are shown in (1) and (2):

(1) BOY SOME FUNNY [ISL]
boy some be.funny
'Some boys are funny/some funny boys […]'

(2) EAMON-HAYES HAPPY [ISL]
Eamon-Hayes be.happy
'Eamon-Hayes was happy/[The] happy Eamon-Hayes […]'

While most signs for these property concepts cannot be inflected for person like verbs (FUNNY and HAPPY are examples of this), others can. Some of these signs have been mentioned in the literature (cf. RIGHT and WRONG in Ó Baoill & Matthews 2000). These property concepts were then called "adjectives that function as verbs". While it is certainly true that these items denote property concepts from a semantic point of view, I think it is indispensable to clearly distinguish semantics and morphosyntax. Thus, from a morphosyntactic point of view, these signs are inflected like verbs and function as predicates. From a syntactic point of view they are, therefore, predicates. This issue is discussed in more detail below.

Another problematic point is the influence from spoken English on ISL resulting in many of the property attributing items preceding the N. Constructions like (3) and (4) were frequent in the data. Generally it can be stated that there are two different construction types that look alike on the surface level. There are either postpositioned attributes (status-assigning predicates) or predicatively used/ property-assigning predicates (Kutscher 2007).

(3)	FABULOUS	PLATE	m.a.t.	[ISL]
	be.fabulous	plate	mat	
	'a fabulous plate mat'			

(4)	DIFFERENT	PART	COUNTRY++	[ISL]
	be.different	part	country.PL	
	'different parts of the country'			

Other influences from spoken English were sometimes visible when spatial syntax was expressed by using English prepositions or by using inflectional or derivational endings from English. Sentences that openly displayed influences from spoken English or another sign language (such as BSL) were also excluded from the analysis. Examples of English morphology that is taken over into ISL can be seen in (5) and (6).[83]

(5) THEY NEED ME BAD **–LY** [ISL]
'They need me badly.'

(6) MOTHER [...] DRINK-TEA **–ING** TEA [ISL]
'The mother was drinking tea.'

In (5), the English inflectional ending for adverbs is used, in (6) the English inflectional ending for the progressive. The signs, taken over from Signed

English, are in fact homonymous signs that look the same for both inflectional endings although different meanings are expressed in the different contexts.

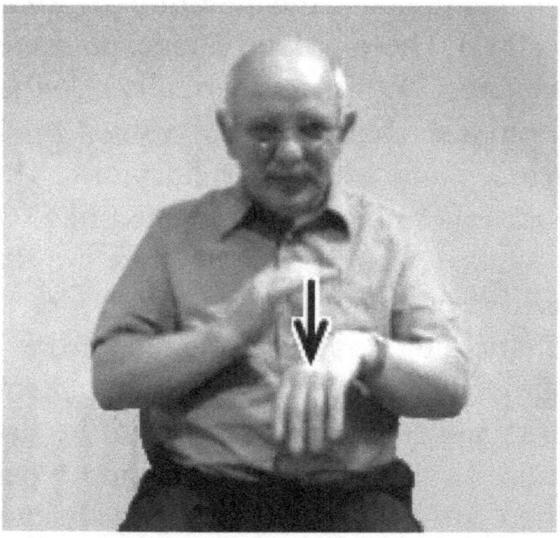

Figure 6.1 Inflectional ending in Signed English

While this phenomenon also had a certain impact on syntax and basic word order, it was especially problematic with respect to category distinguishing morphology for lexical classes. It will be taken up in section 6.2.2.

After the above outline of problematic issues concerning the establishment of syntactic categories in ISL, I will now turn to the syntactic categorization of signs in the data. The category that is most easily and most obviously identified is that of **predicates**. Distributionally, items that are morphologically marked for person (including reflexivity and reciprocity), direction of movement/transfer and optionally aktionsart are restricted to the predicate slot sentence finally.[84] Sentence final predicates thus most frequently show rather complex morphological marking. While these predicates often occur with an explicit argument, they may also occur on their own, i.e. with implicit arguments (cf. Leeson 2001) and constitute the utterance. Examples can be seen in (7) with an explicit argument and (8) with implicit arguments:

(7) CONDUCTOR CL-5-PALM-UP [ISL]
conductor 5.CLtwo-legged-entity.walk-past-speaker
'Five conductors walked past me.'

(8) meet-person++ [ISL]
meet.person.PL
'I met several people.'

As can be seen in (7), classifier predicates always have to be preceded by the referring NP, CONDUCTOR in this case. Non-classificatory agreement verbs like MEET in (8) do not need to fulfill this requirement.[85]

Predicate phrases do not always occur sentence finally though. Especially in sentences including explicit arguments, they are often sentence medial or sometimes even sentence initial. These predicates are usually not marked morphosyntactically, i.e. that the items filling these slots cannot be marked for person and direction of movement/transfer. Optionally, they are marked for aktionsart (intensive, iterative, distributive expressed by reduplication). As they are distributionally and morphosyntactically different from predicate phrases as described above, I suggest a different terminology here. The term **bare predicates** seems appropriate.

Turning to the next syntactic category, arguments are constituted by NPs or **referential phrases**. Similar to bare predicates, they are often morphosyntactically unmarked. However, they can be optionally marked for number and the possessive. Both markings can also be expressed periphrastically. An example of signs restricted to the argument slot is BOY in example (1). It also provides an example of the optionality of number marking which is exclusively expressed by the quantifier SOME. Another option to express number would be by adding a numeral.

Modifier phrases, as mentioned in section 6.2, can either precede or follow NPs. Distributionally, it is thus sometimes difficult to identify them. This is enforced by the fact that they are also optionally marked for aktionsart. However, only intensive and distributive aktionsart are possible in this case whereas they cannot be marked for the iterative. An example of a modifier phrase following a referential phrase is shown in (9). In this case, the slot is morphosyntactically unmarked.

(9)	INDEX+fr	WANT	SHOVEL	GOOD	[ISL]
	1SG	want	shovel	be.good	
	'I want a good shovel.'				

While reduplication of the item GOOD (GOOD++) could either signify an intensive reading, 'very good', or a distributive reading presupposing a plural NP, 'several good shovels', an iterative reading is rather unlikely, *'repeatedly good'. This would rather be expressed periphrastically. Testing for the possibility of iterative reading is therefore a practical tool for the distinction between bare predicate phrases and modifier phrases.

Summarizing the results of this section, it can firstly be stated that ISL possesses four different syntactic categories. These categories including their characteristics are the following:

1. **Predicates**: occur sentence finally, are marked for person or direction of movement/transfer and possibly aktionsart. Example: MEET-PERSON.
2. **Bare predicates**: occur sentence initially, medially and finally, can be optionally marked for intensive, distributive and iterative aktionsart. Example: CRY.
3. **Referential phrases**: syntactically unrestricted, can be optionally marked for number and possessive. Example: BOY.
4. **Modifier phrases**: precede or follow referential phrases, can be optionally marked for intensive and distributive aktionsart. Example: GOOD.

Having outlined the syntactic categories of ISL, I will now turn to the lexical classes of the language. A crucial point of this analysis will be to determine the patterning of lexical classes onto syntactic categories.

6.2.2. Lexical Classes of ISL

Lexical classes, as mentioned frequently in the literature, are not purely based on semantic or ontological criteria (cf. e.g. Sasse 1993a, b). The correlation of formal word classes with conceptual classes has often been used as an additional tool in determining lexical categories though. While it has been proven that conceptual classes exist for all languages, they are by no means the same cross-linguistically (Croft 1991). Sasse (1993a:202) calls "the existence of universal ontological categories a problematic idea, viewed current findings in cognitive linguistics". Ontological criteria will only be one of the minor parameters used for determining the lexical classes of ISL. The ontological classification of ISL lexical items will have to be conducted independent of ontological classifications in other sign languages, English or Irish.

A more important parameter for the determination of lexical classes is morphology. As in the above section on syntactic categories, I have exclusively considered content words in this analysis. However, it can be stated that there seems to be a larger class of functional particles in ISL that includes prepositions and pronouns/indexicals, for instance. All these items have in common that they are under no circumstances morphologically markable while content words can occur with morphological markers.

Most easily identifiable from a morphological point of view is the class of **full verbs**. The verb itself constitutes a lexical base that has to be marked for person or direction of movement/transfer when inserted into a sentence. They are thus closely linked to spatial syntax and reference points in the signing space. This lexical class coincides with the syntactic category of predicates, examples are sentences (7) and (8) in the previous section. From an ontological point of view, these verbs are always dynamic verbs and never stative. They usually refer to some sort of action involving movement in space, literally or metaphorically.[86] One group of signs that seems to be problematic in this respect is all signs denoting conversational acts such as TELL or ASK. Although their morphological properties are the same as those of the other members of the verb class, their semantics do not seem to involve an action of movement. I suggest that the (metaphorical) movement component of these signs is expressed very clearly in the visual-gestural modality. To be more precise, it is an action of transfer that is performed. The item that is transferred here is the verbal message (from speaker to addressee or vice versa in so called backwards verbs[87]). This message is visually represented by the hand configuration that moves from speaker to addressee (cf. figure 2.7). It is the visual-gestural modality that makes us realize the inherent semantics of these kinds of verbs. Therefore, it is legitimate to categorize them as verbs from a morphological as well as from an ontological/semantic point of view.

While most studies on verbs in sign languages refer to Padden's (1988) tripartite classification of the verb class into plain verbs, agreement verbs and spatial verbs, I found this not to be applicable to the data from the SOI. Generally and independent of the ISL data, the distinction seems to be a semantic instead of a morphosyntactic one. Aronoff et al. (2005) mention that spatial verbs denote motion in space, while agreement verbs denote transfer and plain verbs neither nor. From a morphosyntactic point of view, spatial verbs are said to have beginning and end points determined by their spatial referents, while agreement verbs have beginning and end points determined by the referential loci of their arguments, and plain verbs have invariant beginning and end points. However, the distinction between spatial referents and referential loci (which are ultimately also just certain spatial reference points) seems to be rather marginal. Apart from the arguments against the distinction between spatial and agreement verbs mentioned in this paragraph, the literature on ISL does not support this distinction either. Ó Baoill and Matthews (2000) mention only two verbal subclasses: **morphologically marked** and **morphologically unmarked verbs**. Consequently, the dichotomous distinction of morphologically marked verbs into spatial and agreement verbs does not seem plausible and is not further applied for the current study.

The subclass of plain verbs suggested by Padden does not seem plausible from a syntactic point of view for the ISL data either. Many items of an alleged plain verb category occur with predicative function, however, these predicates are not sentence final in transitive sentences. This is in line with Leeson's (2001) statement that basic clause structure in transitive sentences including "plain verbs" is theme-verb-undergoer (including explicit arguments), while it is theme-verb(-undergoer) (with possible implicit arguments) in sentences featuring a morphologically marked verb. Viewed these facts, what has been traditionally called "plain verbs" do not belong to the main class of full verbs but form a lexical class of their own. Additionally, they do not show the same morphosyntactic features as full verbs, as they cannot be inflected for person or direction of movement/transfer. However, they can be optionally marked for aktionsart (iterative, intensive, distributive). Examples of this kind of lexical item are shown in (10) to (12).

(10)	HAVE	BANANA	BOAT				[ISL]
	have	banana	boat				
	'[We] had a banana boat.'						

(11)	r.d.s.	AFTER	INDEX+f	STOP	FOR	CUP-OF-TEA	[ISL]
	rds	after	LOC	stop	for	cup.tea	
	'After the RDS (there), we stopped for a cup of tea.'						

(12)	LAST	DAY	INDEX+sr	CRY++	[ISL]
	last	day	1PL	cry.INT	
	'The last day we cried a lot.'				

Sentence (10) shows a transitive sentence with a sentence initial predicate. HAVE in ISL cannot be marked for person, a marking for direction of movement/transfer is not possible due to the inherent semantics of the item. It also could not be marked for aktionsart. Example (11) shows an intransitive context with an alleged plain verb. Similar to the previous example, it could neither be marked for person nor for direction of movement/transfer. However, it could be marked for iterative aktionsart expressed by reduplication of the sign. Finally, in sentence (12) CRY is marked for the intensive. Thus the meaning 'to cry a lot' is acquired. Given these morphological characteristics, the signs cannot be classified as full verbs. As aktionsart inflections play a major role in the determination of this class, I termed it **aktionsart verbs 1**.

Moreover, property concepts as mentioned in examples (1) and (2) show similar distributional and morphosyntactic characteristics as aktionsart verbs 1. Most frequently, they occur as heads of predicates and they cannot be inflected for person or direction of movement/transfer either. These signs often occur as heads of predicates but might, as opposed to aktionsart verbs 1, occur as heads of modifiers (attributively). In the past, this has led researchers to state that these signs are adjectives. This conclusion seems to be based on additional semantic criteria (the items denoting property concepts) and seems biased by the researchers' mother tongues (English or other European languages) in which property concepts are expressed by a class of adjectives (cf. Sasse 1993a:202). In ISL it seems that these items rather have to be interpreted as stative verbs. Hellwig (2010) discusses a similar problem for Goemai (a West Chadic language of the Afroasiatic language phylum). Viewed the features outlined in the previous paragraph, a syntactic category of adjectives seems unlikely for ISL. Rather, items of the kind exemplified in sentences (1), (2), (9) and (13) seem to belong to the class of aktionsart verbs. The first three examples do not show inflection for aktionsart though. Only in (13) reduplication representing intensive aspect is shown. Despite this one very straightforward example, it is not always clear whether the reduplication of movement that expresses aktionsart might not actually be a distributive marker. Consider SAME++ in the following context:

(13)	EVERY DAY	DIFFERENT++ [...]	OFFICE [...]	SAME++	[ISL]
	everyday	be.different.DISTR	office	be.same.INT	

'[At school] every day is different. In an office it's very much the same.'

While the transcription suggests an intensive interpretation, it could very well be a marker for the distributive, taking up the distributive marker of DIFFERENT++. It turns out that only in the cases involving an aspectual sign, the distributive marker can be excluded. In all other cases, a distributive reading is as possible as an intensive one and can only be inferred from the (syntactic) context. This in itself is reason enough to distinguish a separate lexical class. While being similar to aktionsart verbs 1 in terms of general patterning, some distributional criteria (additional occurrence in modifier slots instead of referential phrases) and some morphological criteria (no inflection for iterative) are different from items in this category. Consequently, I subcategorized the class and called the first group **aktionsart verbs 1** and the latter **aktionsart verbs 2**.

A further lexical class that could be determined is morphologically recognizable by optional marking for number and the possessive. The exact dynamics of this marking were already mentioned in section 6.2.1, showing that this marking does not have to take place by morphological inflection but can be expressed periphrastically using quantifiers or pronouns. Examples could be seen in most sentences, such as BOY in (1), MOTHER in (6) or SHOVEL in (9). Syntactically, these items are restricted to referential phrases. The class includes mostly signs that can precede a classificatory verb as head of an NP. Often, but not exclusively, these signs function as subjects. This class of items is referred to as **nouns**.

Apart from signs like aktionsart verbs 2 that can occur in two different syntactic slots, there are a few signs that are even less syntactically specified. These items can occur as heads of predicates, as heads of attributive modifiers and as heads of referential phrases. Examples of these are the signs HEARING or DEAF, of which the latter is shown in sentences (14) – (16).

(14) ONE DEAF SAY CURIOUS INDEX+f,hi [ISL]
one deaf say be.curious 3SG
'One deaf person said he was curious.'

(15) [...] WITH FRIEND FOUR DEAF PERSON [ISL]
with friend four be.deaf person
'[...] with four deaf friends.'

(16) INDEX+me DEAF [ISL]
1SG be.deaf
'I am deaf.'

In (14), DEAF is the head of the argument, whereas it functions as attributive modifier in (15). In (16), it is the head of the predicate. As can be seen in the examples, no category changing morphology is needed in order to make the sign available for another syntactic category. However, it is possible to morphologically mark items like DEAF or HEARING for all morphological categories except for person and direction of movement/transfer. This morphological as well as syntactic indeterminacy results in a high degree of multifunctionality. This is in line with current sign linguistic theory postulating that due to their young age sign languages exhibit a rather large number of multifunctional categories (Meir 2012). I call this lexical class **multifunctional signs**. While Erlenkamp (2000) categorized all DGS signs other than verbs as multifunctional signs with different sub-classes, signs like DEAF or HEARING display the utmost degree of multifunctionality in ISL. Accordingly, when referring to "multifunctional signs" in this book, only signs that can fill argument, predicate and modifier slots are referred to.[88]

After this general outline of the morphological and syntactic criteria determining the different lexical classes of ISL, I will briefly turn to the semantic/ontological criterion. Regarding the class of full verbs it was already mentioned that semantically, all items belonging to this class denote some kind of transfer or motion in space. This might also be realized metaphorically (cf. the beginning of this section).

Concerning aktionsart verbs, these signs are not clearly identifiable as a class on semantic ontological grounds. Even within the subclasses of aktionsart verbs 1 and 2, items tend to vary in their meaning. In order for the expressed notions of aktionsart verbs 1 to be available for iterative aspect, many of them have a dynamic and a telic component as non-telic items usually seem weird in iterative contexts. Examples of this are BUY, END, HURRY and STOP. With respect to the subclass of aktionsart verbs 2, it seems that they constitute a class of property concepts. However, it has become clear from the examples and the rest of the data that an interpretation as stative verbs seems more adequate.

Finally turning to nouns, the items of this class refer to objects, individuals, abstract concepts and states. The semantics of this class thus seem relatively homogeneous.

Summarizing the results obtained in this section, there are four main lexical classes of ISL signs. These classes, including their morphological, syntactic and semantic features, are shown below.

1. **Full verbs**: morphologically marked for person and direction of movement/transfer, occur in sentence final predicates only, are usually dynamic verbs denoting (metaphorical) movement in space. Example: MEET-PERSON.
2. **Aktionsart verbs 1**: morphologically markable for intensive or iterative aktionsart, occur in sentence initial, medial and final bare predicates, many involve a telic meaning component. Example: CRY.
   Aktionsart verbs 2: morphologically markable for distributive and intensive aktionsart, occur in sentence initial, medial and final bare predicates and modifiers, denote property concepts or "stative verbs". Example: FUNNY.
3. **Nouns**: morphologically markable for number and possessive, occur in referential phrases only, denote objects, individuals, abstract concepts or states. Example: BOY.
4. **Multifunctional signs**: morphologically markable for everything but person and direction of movement/transfer, occur in all syntactic categories but (full) predicates, semantically indeterminate. Example: DEAF.

While the number of lexical classes is the same as that of syntactic categories, they are not congruent. The class of lexical full verbs coincides with the syntactic predicate slot, just as aktionsart verbs 1 always fill the bare predicate slot and the lexical class of nouns coincides with referential phrases. However, the class of aktionsart verbs 2 can fill bare predicate as well as modifier slots and multifunctional signs can fill every syntactic slot except that of predicates.

Altogether, ISL turned out to be a TYPE B language according to Sasse's (1993a) classification: while both syntactic categories and lexical classes can be distinguished, they do not match. Figure 6.2 below shows the relations between the syntactic categories and the lexical classes of ISL. As this was commented on extensively in the above analysis, the component of the morphological form of the sign is not shown in Figure 6.2.

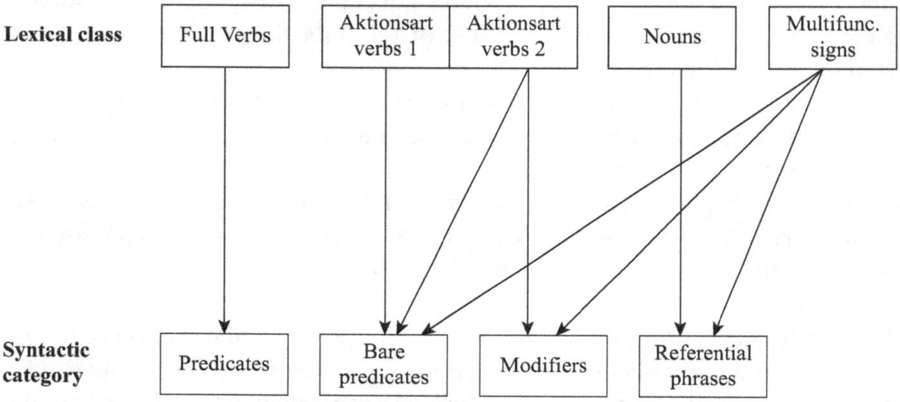

Figure 6.2 Relation of lexical classes and syntactic categories in ISL

After having distinguished the lexical classes of ISL and compared them to the syntactic categories established in the previous section, I will now take a closer look at the question whether mouth actions can be used as a modality specific tool for word class recognition in ISL. In order to do so, the next section investigates the correlations of the ISL word classes with the different types of mouth actions.

6.2.3. Correlations of Word Classes and Mouth Actions

As mentioned at the beginning of this chapter, it has been previously stated that there seems to be a correlation between the different kinds of mouth actions and word classes in sign languages. This correlation is ultimately based on the parameter of morphological complexity as mentioned in 6. Thus, other researchers found morphologically less complex signs to correlate with mouthings while morphologically complex structures frequently occurred with mouth gestures. However, in most cases, syntactic categories and lexical classes as the basis of the analysis were conflated, due to parameters from different levels that were applied and not properly distinguished. The case of the morphosyntactic tripartite verb distinction by Padden (1988) often applied without further investigation is only one example. Consequently, earlier findings with respect to the correlation of mouth actions and word classes in sign languages can only be a rough guideline for the current investigation.

Having criticized the lack of distinction between syntactic categories and lexical classes in other studies, I clearly want to separate both levels of analysis here. In a first step, the correlation of mouth actions and syntactic categories will be tackled, while the co-occurrences between mouth actions and lexical classes are treated in the second part of this section. Below, the correlation between mouth actions and the syntactic categories of ISL established in chapter 6.2.1 is shown. While the analysis in chapter 5.3 and 5.4 included the category "nothing" besides mouthings and mouth gestures, this has not been included in the investigation of correlation with word classes. With respect to syntactic categories and lexical classes I am exclusively interested in their co-occurrence with mouth actions as this is assumed to correlate with the morphological complexity of a sign. For the sociolinguistic analysis, signs not accompanied by any mouth action were relevant as they hinted at the educational background of a signer, which is why I included the category there.

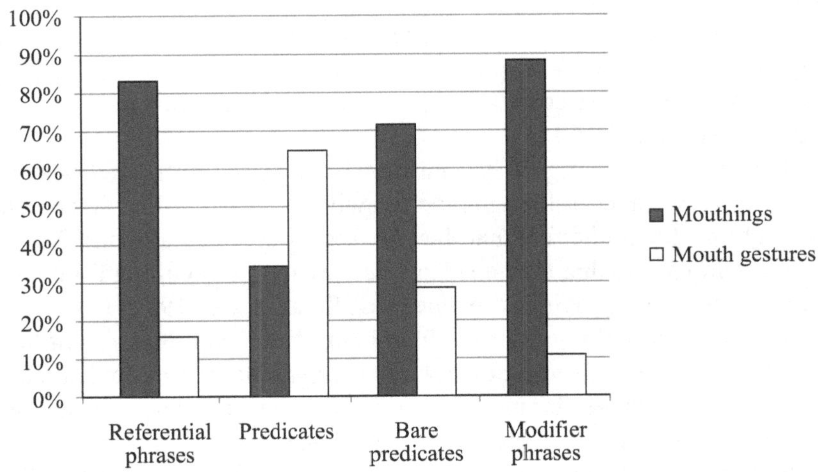

Figure 6.3 Correlation between mouth actions and syntactic categories in ISL

As can be seen in figure 6.3 above, all syntactic categories except for predicates mainly co-occur with mouthings. This was to be expected, given that predicates are the only category with obligatory morphosyntactic marking in ISL. With all other categories, although morphosyntactic marking is possible, it is optional. This is reflected by the figures obtained for co-occurrences with mouth actions. Predicates, on the other hand, have to occur with mouth gestures as they are always morphologically complex in that they have to be inflected for a spatial morpheme.

Despite the fact that bare predicates, referential phrases and modifiers all co-occur most frequently with mouthings, subtle differences between the frequencies are visible. Referential phrases show high frequencies of co-occurrence with mouthings (83.7% = 246 items), modifiers even higher (89.1% = 49 items). Bare predicates are slightly different from these two categories as they occur less frequently with mouthings (71.6% = 240 items). This indicates their higher morphosyntactic complexity as compared to the other two categories. It also hints at the fact that morphological marking is more frequent (although also optional) with this category than with the others. However, altogether it can be stated that all investigated categories occur most frequently with mouthings, except for predicates which occur most frequently with mouth gestures (65.6% = 118 items).

Given these findings, mouth actions do not seem to be a very helpful tool in the determination of a sign's syntactic category in ISL. They may only serve to make a major distinction between predicates and all other syntactic categories. A slot correlating with a mouth gesture is often a predicate, but a slot accompanied by a mouthing might be a referential phrase, a bare predicate or a modifier phrase.

Having looked at the co-occurrence of mouth actions with the syntactic categories of ISL, I will now turn to the lexical classes of the language. Figure 6.4 displays the correlation between mouth actions and the lexical classes of ISL established in section 6.2.2.

When looking at the figure it seems noteworthy that multifunctional signs are the category that correlates most often with mouthings (85.7% = 6 items). This might be due to the fact that they are highly semantically and functionally indeterminate so that they need an accompanying mouthing for meaning disambiguation. This claim is in line with Schermer's (1990) paradigm of the functions of mouthings, one of them being the disambiguation of homonyms. As can be seen from figure 6.4, the results obtained for lexical classes are also similar to those obtained for syntactic categories. The morphological complexity of signs is reflected in these co-occurrences in that mouthings frequently occur with nouns which are morphologically less complex (due to

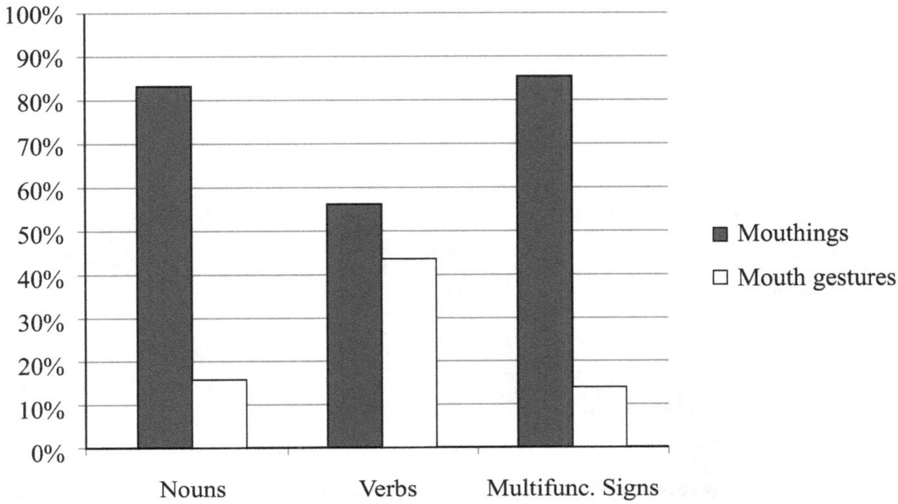

Figure 6.4 Correlation between lexical classes and mouth actions in ISL

optional morphological marking) than verbs. The latter frequently co-occur with mouth gestures (43.7% = 257 items) which is in line with the hypothesis set up earlier. It should also be mentioned that compounds, which were mentioned in 6, always occurred with mouthings. This exclusively refers to compound structures that are also found in spoken languages, such as noun + noun. An example of this could be seen in (3) where both parts PLATE and m.a.t. were accompanied by mouthings. Dvandva compounds were not found in the data and can therefore not be commented on. Concerning the sub-classification of the verb class, the general split between full verbs and aktionsart verbs is clearly visible in the co-occurrences with mouth actions. The distinction between aktionsart verbs 1 and 2 is hardly visible though, frequencies of co-occurrence with mouth gestures are very similar (73% = 197 items with mouthings in aktionsart verbs 1, 71.3% (72 items) with mouthings in aktionsart verbs 2). This is illustrated again in figure 6.5.

While at a first glance this seems to question the sub-classification of aktionsart verbs into 1 and 2, there are enough arguments in favour of this distinction. One of the reasons for distinguishing two different subclasses was distribution. This however, is not reflected by co-occurrences with mouth actions. Moreover, while the morphology and morphosyntax of aktionsart verbs 1 and 2 is different in quality, i.e. different kinds of aktionsart are applicable, it is not different in complexity. As co-occurrences with mouth gestures only reflect the morphological complexity of a sign, no significant distinction is visible between aktionsart verbs 1 and 2 in this respect.

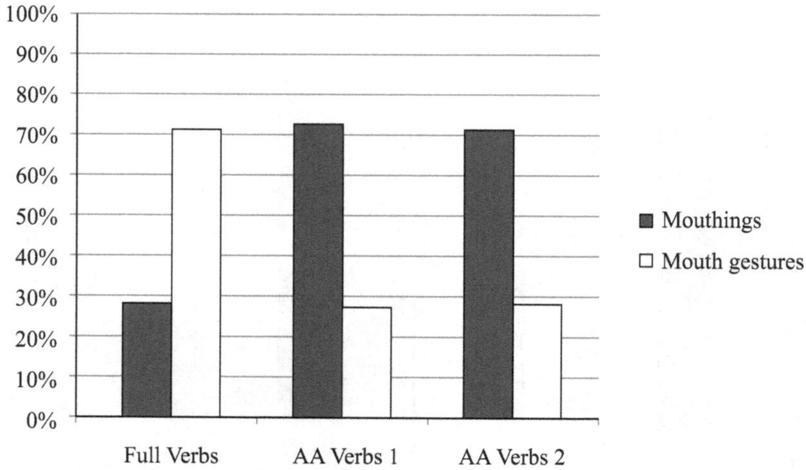

Figure 6.5 Correlations between mouth actions and verbal sub-classes in ISL

In summary, the larger sub-classification of the verb class is reflected by co-occurrences with mouth actions, for a more fine-grained sub-categorization, morphological and distributional criteria are necessary.

Summarizing the results of this section, it can be concluded that the hypothesis that morphologically complex signs frequently co-occur with mouth gestures while morphologically simpler structures correlate with mouthings could be proven. However, no fine-grained distinction between the different syntactic categories and lexical classes of ISL can be achieved by looking at mouth actions only. They solely reflect the split between morphologically very complex full verbs/predicates and morphologically simpler structures. I also want to distance myself from earlier claims that mouth actions indicate or correlate with certain word classes. This does not seem to be the case, at least not in ISL. Consequently, and contrary to claims made by other researchers, analyzing correlations between mouth actions and word classes in ISL is no practical modality-specific tool for word class recognition or establishment. The most salient parameters for the distinction of syntactic categories and lexical classes are distribution and morphology, mouth actions merely hint at the morphological complexity of an item.

6.2.4. Mouth Gestures as a Category in Its Own Right?

The last issue that seems noteworthy in the context of word classes in ISL is mouth gestures. This might seem rather odd, given that mouth gestures were already treated in the previous section on correlations between syntactic categories/lexical classes and mouth actions. However, a certain feature of mouth gestures that has been observed for different sign languages was also found for the ISL data. This feature is the iconicity of certain mouth gestures and it is the iconicity of these mouth gestures combined with their distributional properties that attracted my attention. Before analyzing the ISL data with respect to this point however, a short summary of the literature on the iconicity of mouth gestures and the iconic word class of ideophones, found in many Asian and African languages, will be provided.

Sandler (2009) commented on the phenomenon of iconic mouth gestures in IsSL, Fischer and Kollien (2009) on DGS, Fowler and Heaton (2006) on BSL and Woll (2001) (although from a slightly different angle) also on BSL. In her article on the symbiotic relation between hand and mouth in sign languages in general and in IsSL in particular, Sandler argued that there is a certain type of mouth gesture that is gestural in nature as it is not conventionalized and subject to idiosyncracies of signers. Moreover, these mouth gestures all seem to be iconic. She defined iconic gestures along the lines of theories from gesture studies (McNeill 1992; Kendon 2004) as "gestures that picture aspects of the object or event being described by speech. [... They] create a likeness of an object or concept symbolically, through a configuration of the hands (or mouth)" (Sandler 2009:249ff). She clearly distinguishes these gestures from lexical material and explicitly mentions that not all mouth gestures belong to this category. Conventionalized adjectival and adverbial mouth gestures do not form part of her object of study. The most important points of her analysis are that although non-standard, these mouth gestures contribute to the overall meaning of an utterance (hence the term symbiosis) and they often occur with classifier predicates.

Fischer and Kollien (2009) also distinguished between different kinds of mouth gestures and commented on those that are iconic in nature. These iconic kinds of mouth gestures mostly seem to occur with highly idiomatic sign language utterances and classifier constructions. The overall question they tried to answer in their study was whether onomatopoeia exist in DGS and whether they are expressed by mouth gestures. They argued, similarly to Sandler, that mouth gestures add to the semantic content of an utterance. According to them, constructed action, classifier constructions and onomatopoeic mouth gestures all add to the meaning of a proposition and result in the immense complexity of sign language utterances. Answering their research question they found that sounds are not expressed iconically by mouth gestures, i.e. that there was no proof for onomatopoeia in a narrow sense in DGS.[89] However, they made another interesting finding. Many of the iconic mouth gestures are visualizations of other sensory qualities (esp. tactile qualities in their experiments). They called the use of mouth gestures in this context the "synaesthetic symbolisation of tactile perception" (Fischer & Kollien 2009:466).

The theory of echo phonology was already outlined in detail in section 3.4.2. The important issue to be mentioned here is that the other studies outlined in this section focused on non-conventionalized mouth gestures and their iconicity related to the extra-linguistic world. Woll's echo phonology analyzed mainly conventionalized mouth gestures that are iconic in that they depict the manual sign on the mouth. Moreover, these mouth gestures are obligatory for the manual sign to be well formed. This contradicts the abovementioned theories in that they emphasize the fact that only non-conventionalized mouth gestures are iconic. A point which all studies agree upon is that (conventionalized) adverbial mouth gestures are usually not iconic. However, I will try to show that this is not the case (in ISL).

In fact, I want to argue that certain mouth gestures might even form a category in its own right. All of the mouth gestures in question are iconic, either in the way described by Sandler (2009), Fischer and Kollien (2009) or by Woll (2001). As these mouth gestures also mainly occur with certain manual sign structures, they seem similar to a word class abundant in many languages of Asia and Africa, namely ideophones. A brief introduction to ideophones is provided in the following.

Ideophones have not received very much attention in word class research as they tend to occur in the more "exotic" languages of the world and are elusive with respect to grammar. They are usually absent from sample sentences as they are difficult to elicit. While terminology suggests some kind of relation to sound and it might therefore be weird to mention them in the context of sign languages that are situated in the visual-gestural modality, newer studies on ideophones emphasize their general relation to all kinds of sensory imagery. "Ideophones are marked words that depict sensory imagery" (Dingemanse 2011), "[...] ideophones are expressives, characterising sounds, sensations, textures and feelings, usually but not always, through morphological patterning" (Blench 2009). This is shown in examples from Bura (a Chadic language spoken in Nigeria): *bádábádá*= 'describes running fast', *cipcip*= 'in good order, straight, orderly' and *curr* = 'describes the sound of water pouring into a vessel' (Blench 2004). Only the last of these examples is concerned with sound symbolism, while the other two actually describe other sensory imagery.

As could be seen from the definitions and examples, ideophones are very much concerned with iconicity in language in that they depict sensory imagery by linguistic means. While they do so by using sounds in spoken languages, I suggest that there is a similar phenomenon in sign languages which expresses this sensory imagery by mouth gestures. Another characteristic of ideophones noteworthy at this point is their markedness. These words are marked by clearly standing out phonotactically and morphologically from other words of a certain language (Dingemanse 2011). Moreover, their meanings are usually difficult to describe as they are at the centre of idiomatic expressions of a language. Their etymology is usually rather hazy (Blench 2009). Ideophones are usually not restricted to one specific lexical class of a language. However, there is a certain tendency to occur in the adverb or verb class in African languages (Westermann 1907; Blench 2009), a fact that is not surprising, viewed that it is often actions that are depicted. They are clearly conventionalized forms and are not made up ad hoc, depending on the context of a situation. Nevertheless, new ideophones are invented as new technologies are introduced to societies (Blench 2009). Keeping these core characteristics in mind, I will now turn to the investigation of a subgroup of mouth gestures in ISL.

Having distinguished three different kinds of mouth gestures (semantically empty, enacting and adverbial mouth gestures) in section 3.4.1, it is almost obvious that only two of these kinds of mouth gestures can be considered in the context of ideophones, namely adverbial and enacting mouth gestures. As the class of ideophones is usually easily identifiable semantically (Blench 2009), semantically empty mouth gestures are excluded from the analysis. Consequently, it seemed most sensible to exclusively look at mouth gestures occurring with lexical verbs (either full or aktionsart). Mouth actions that fulfilled these criteria (belonging either to the category of enacting or adverbial mouth gestures and hence occurring with a manual verb) show a striking degree of iconicity. One very good example of this was shown in figure 4.14 (again shown for convenience in figure 6.6), exemplifying PLAY-HARD-AGAINST-EACH-OTHER.

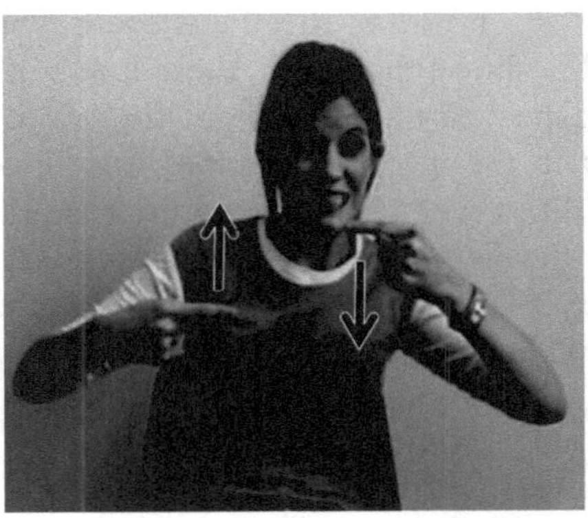

Figure 6.6 The ISL sign PLAY-HARD-AGAINST-EACH-OTHER

The adverb 'hard' is expressed by the clenched teeth mouth gesture. This mouth gesture is iconic in that it depicts an action that a person could exhibit in a fight or a serious game like the one reported in the story. Moreover, it also fits the movement of the hands which is strained and slower than in the sign unmodified by an adverbial. Figure 4.17 (again shown in 6.7), depicting THROW-DOWN-SHOVEL (angrily), also provides a good example of an iconic mouth gesture.

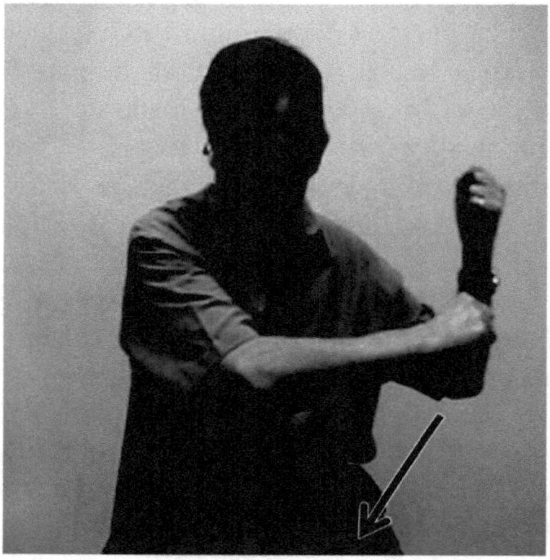

Figure 6.7 The ISL sign THROW-DOWN-SHOVEL

Although the adverb is not expressed in the gloss, this is a problem of transcription, as it is clearly taken up by the following verb STORM-OFF. The closed, stretched mouth is iconic in that it depicts the deep exhaling one would actually display when in anger and lips pressed together angrily, while on a second level it reflects the downward movement of the manual sign. This shows that while these kinds of mouth gestures are often iconic with respect to the extralinguistic world, they might also be iconic with respect to the manual sign they accompany. This is a point made by Woll (2001) as well. It might be the case that a high degree of lexical iconicity in the verb sign enforces this phenomenon as it can be observed for THROW-DOWN-SHOVEL, reminiscent of a pantomimic movement. Apart from the adverbial mouth gestures, enacting mouth gestures are often iconic as well. Figure 4.23 (again shown in 6.8), depicting the sign CALL, is obviously iconic with respect to the action of calling from the extralinguistic world.

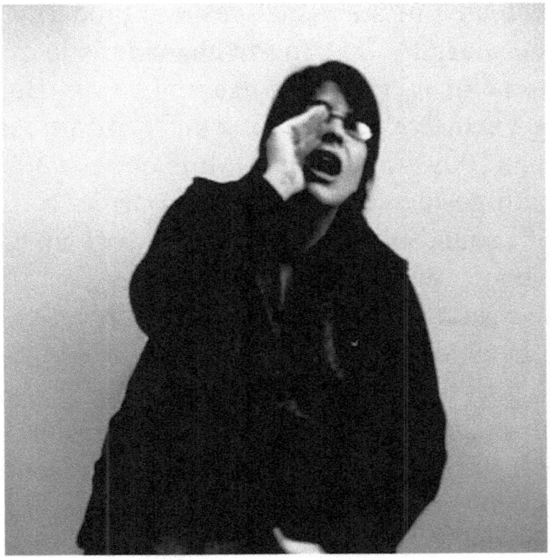

Figure 6.8 The ISL sign CALL

As this mouth gesture constitutes the whole sign, it cannot be iconic concerning the action of the hands. This sign seems to be extremely marked in that it only involves a limited manual component. A similar example is the sign LICK (figure 4.21) which sometimes lacked the manual component. However, if it included a manual sign, the mouth gesture can be said to be iconic on two different levels, one depicting the action of licking in the extra-linguistic world, the other reflecting the movement of the hands iconically depicting the licking action.

Applying Dingemanse's (2011) definition of ideophones to the above-mentioned examples of mouth gestures in ISL, a class of ideophones seems reasonable. The first criterion of his definition, markedness, was already mentioned briefly above. Structurally, iconic mouth gestures are extremely marked as compared to other lexical classes in that they only use one of the articulators available in sign languages (the mouth), in order to convey meaning. This is especially the case with respect to adverbial mouth gestures that accompany manual signs. Enacting mouth gestures might be even more marked as they can constitute the whole sign (verb), lacking a manual component altogether. The criterion of being a word of the respective language is slightly more complicated than the other criteria and will thus be treated at the end of this outline.

Turning to the feature of depiction, it is evident that mouth gestures depict the extralinguistic world or the manual component in an iconic way. The term depiction actually applies in a very literal sense in this case, as mouth gestures are also situated in the visual-gestural modality and can therefore visually depict their meaning. The fourth characteristic of ideophones refers to expressing sensory imagery. In the examples from Bura it became clear that this does not exclusively refer to sounds. Additionally, the study by Fischer and Kollien (2009) showed that while onomatopoeia do not seem to exist in DGS, mouth gestures often iconically depict tactile feelings. In the examples from ISL, sounds as well as other sensory imagery were depicted iconically. CALL iconically depicts sound imagery, while LICK and HARD refer to the tactile sense. THROW-DOWN-SHOVEL is really an action and thus similar to *bádábádá* which also describes an action or a certain movement.

Finally returning to the issue of ideophones being words, it is not clear whether this criterion actually refers to mouth gestures in ISL. As was mentioned earlier in this book, there are certainly some mouth gestures that are conventionalized, always occurring in the same form with the same meaning (e.g. the manner markers of ISL). However, there is a large number of mouth gestures that are non-conventionalized. Some of them were included in the examples mentioned above (e.g. THROW-DOWN-SHOVEL with a closed, stretched down mouth gesture). They could not be considered words as this would imply a conventionalization component and these mouth gestures are clearly not part of the lexicon of ISL. Despite this fact I would argue for their inclusion in an ideophone class.

In conclusion, I suggest another lexical class of ISL signs, namely that of ideophones expressed exclusively on the mouth. Distributionally, they usually occur with verbs or constitute a "verb" themselves.[90] So far, mouth gestures have been neglected with respect to word class research in sign languages – or rather, they have been considered a modality-specific tool for the distinction of word classes. However, I propose that apart from that, they are a category in its own right that requires further investigation.

6.2.5. Discussion of the Results within a Functional Linguistic Model

The first part of this chapter was exclusively concerned with the theoretical background of word class research, including its historical development from the Ancient Greeks to present-day typological approaches and theories on word class distinctions in sign languages. This outline showed that the idea of categorizing the world or language according to human cognition reaches back to antiquity. However, the categorizations applied to languages such as Ancient Greek or Latin were often too readily and incorrectly applied to other languages. Moreover, many studies exclusively considered one of the many criteria that are necessary for a thorough distinction of word classes, concentrating solely on morphology, syntax, semantics or discourse-pragmatics. It was emphasized that all these factors need to be combined in order to achieve a plausible parts-of-speech distinction. Although the parameters applied are universal, parts-of-speech classifications are always language specific. A final point made in this context was that syntactic categories and lexical classes have to be distinguished in present day theories and that languages constitute one of four types according to the matching of their syntactic categories with their lexical classes. Most Indo-European languages constitute TYPE A languages in which syntactic categories and lexical classes coincide, a fact that has led researchers to believe for a long time that all languages function according to this pattern. Concerning theories on PoS distinctions in sign languages, it was stated that to date, word class research in sign languages, especially from a typological point of view, has been rather neglected. Most researchers simply applied the PoS distinction from their native spoken language to the investigated sign language. For many sign languages, different movement patterns between nouns and verbs have been claimed. A tripartite morphosyntactic distinction of the verb class has been claimed for most sign languages, ignoring the fact that this distinction was originally developed for ASL and is based on ASL syntax. Finally, co-occurrences of certain word classes with mouth actions have been claimed for many sign languages, generally based on differences in the morphological setup of the respective signs. The overall argument was that morphologically complex signs co-occur with mouth gestures while morphologically simple signs coincide with mouthings.

In the second part of this chapter, the ISL data were analyzed regarding PoS distinctions. It was found that on the syntactic level, there are four different syntactic categories distinguished by their distribution and morphosyntax. Predicates always occur sentence finally and are always morphologically marked for person or direction of movement/ transfer. Bare predicates occur sentence initially, medially and finally and are optionally marked for aktionsart. Referential phrases are syntactically unrestricted and are optionally marked for number and/or possessive. Modifier phrases precede or follow referential phrases and are optionally marked for aktionsart. With respect to the lexical classes of ISL, it was firstly found that the traditional tripartite distinction of the verb class as claimed by Padden (1988) for ASL does not apply to ISL. The lexical class of verbs is sub-classified into two categories, full verbs and aktionsart verbs which can in turn be sub-classified into aktionsart verbs 1 and 2. Generally, there are four different lexical classes in ISL, distinguished on morphological grounds. Full verbs are morphologically marked for person or direction of movement/transfer. Aktionsart verbs 1 are optionally marked for iterative and intensive aktionsart while aktionsart verbs 2 are optionally marked for intensive and distributive aktionsart. Nouns are optionally marked for number and/or possessive. Multifunctional signs are morphologically markable for every morphological category except for person and direction of movement/transfer.

When analyzing the matching of syntactic categories and lexical classes, it turned out that ISL is a TYPE B language in Sasse's (1993a) terminology, in which both syntactic categories and lexical classes can be distinguished but do not coincide. Accordingly, full verbs are restricted to the predicate slot, aktionsart verbs 1 to the bare predicate slot and nouns to referential phrases. Aktionsart verbs 2 are syntactically multifunctional in that they can occur in bare predicates and modifier phrases. Multifunctional signs are even more syntactically indeterminate, given that they can occur in referential phrases, bare predicates and modifier phrases.

After the establishment of the syntactic categories and lexical classes of ISL, their correlation with mouth actions was tested. The aim of this analysis was to find out whether mouth actions function as a modality-specific tool in word class recognition in ISL. The hypothesis that morphologically simpler signs (nouns/RPs and multifunctional signs/RPs/bare predicates/modifiers) co-occur with mouthings while morphologically complex signs (verbs/predicates) co-occur with mouth gestures, was proven. Moreover, the subclassification of the verb class into full verbs that are highly morphologically complex and aktionsart verbs that are less so, was supported. This however partly refutes the claim that mouth actions serve as a modality-specific tool for word class recognition in ISL, as only the class of full verbs is clearly singled out by its co-occurrence with mouth gestures. All other classes co-occur with mouthings and distributional and morphological criteria are the most salient features for the distinction between the different syntactic categories and lexical classes of ISL.

Finally, it was suggested that mouth gestures might form a category in its own right, namely that of ideophones. This argument is based on the findings with respect to the iconicity of mouth gestures in other sign languages as well as on research on ideophones in the spoken languages of the world. It was shown that adverbial and enacting mouth gestures in ISL are usually iconic and additionally adhere to modern definitions of ideophones. This would expand the lexical classes of ISL to five. Further research in this area seems necessary.

Finally, the results of the current analysis shall be situated within current linguistic theory on word classes. As the categorization of syntactic categories and lexical classes of ISL is based on the criteria put forth by typological studies on spoken languages (Hopper & Thompson 1984; Schachter 1985; Croft 1991, 2000; Hengeveld 1992; Sasse 1993b; Evans 2000; Hengeveld et al. 2004; Rijkhoff 2007; Himmelmann 2008; Haspelmath 2010), the current study is also situated in a typological functional framework. Assuming a close relation between linguistic typology and linguistic functionalism (Croft 1990), the analysis of ISL PoS is situated in a functional grammatical model such as proposed by Dik ([1989] 1997), for instance. Thus, Dik's theory focuses on communicative competence of a natural language user, emphasizing the function of a linguistic expression in its particular setting (Rauh 2010). Pragmatics plays a major role in this theory, constituting an all-encompassing framework (Dik 1997:8). In the following, similarities between the typological functional approaches discussed in 6.1.1–6.1.3 are outlined and possible adjustments with respect to sign languages are proposed.

While chapters 6.1.1–6.1.3 elaborate on the main semantic, syntactic and morphosyntactic approaches to word class distinction, chapter 6.2 summarizes the four main criteria for the categorization of word classes applied to the ISL data: the formal, distributional, ontological-semantic and discourse-pragmatic parameters. These are also listed in typological studies requesting the balanced use of different linguistic parameters for the establishment of word classes (e.g. Schachter 1985; Sasse 1993a). Moreover, the distinction between open and closed classes as proposed in traditional grammar and by typologists like Schachter (1985) is applied to the ISL data as only open classes or lexical categories were investigated (cf. chapter 6.2.1).

Further, and on a more general level, the typology of mouthings proposed in chapter 4.2.1 is clearly functional and meaning-related. Those are for example TYPE 6a (simultaneous compounds/modifiers) in which the mouthing adds a meaning component. Even types such as 4 (inflected mouthings) which in terminology seem to refer to formal criteria, were shown to serve inherently semantic functions in creating semantic congruence. Pragmatic or discourse-related functions that are mentioned as an all-encompassing framework by Dik (1997), are clearly represented by the metalinguistic functions of TYPE 6c (metalinguistic remarks).

An often discussed question in typological analyses of PoS is that of precategoricality or the hen and egg question of what was there first: constructions or lexically categorized items. This is especially relevant for languages with flexible PoS systems such as Samoan that possess lexical items that can fill each syntactic slot. As mentioned in chapter 6.1.4, due to their young age, sign languages possess many multifunctional items that can be used in several syntactic slots. Erlenkamp (2000) is a case in point, categorizing all DGS signs other than verbs as multifunctional. The multifunctionality of signs was also shown for ISL in chapter 6.2.2 with respect to the lexical category of multifunctional signs.[91] The existence of a category like this also raises the question of pre-categoricality.

"Neo-constructionist approaches" (Baker 2003) like Borer (2005a, b) suggest that items are always pre-categorical in that the specification for a lexical category is a matter of syntax. While this works easily for isolating languages like Chinese which is often cited in Borer's work, studies like Himmelmann (2008) disprove this claim. Himmelmann convincingly shows that Tagalog roots are not always neutral. The same holds true for ISL. While multifunctional signs are syntactically indeterminate as compared with full verbs, for instance, they are by no means neutral. Thus, they are not morphologically markable for person and direction of movement/transfer which precludes them from the predicate slot. Similarly, Himmelmann (2008:286 ff.) showed that not all Tagalog roots are compatible with each morphological specification and are therefore not pre-categorical. Consequently, I argue that the items of the multifunctional class in ISL show a rather high degree of neutrality as compared to the other lexical classes but are by no means pre-categorical.

Finally turning to the functional grammar model proposed by Dik (1997), the current study and its results shall be categorized in this framework. A functional grammar according to Dik (1997) consists of three components: the "Fund" which contains the lexicon consisting of "basic predicates" and "basic terms". The second component forms "complex underlying clause structures" on various layers while the third component consists of "expression rules" ordering clause structures (phonologically) and finally forming linguistic expressions. Figure 6.9 shows a schematic representation of Dik's model (modified from Dik 1989:60).

Viewed this model, Dik argues that the formation of nuclear predications is achieved by combining basic or derived predicates with basic or derived terms from the Fund. Except for basic terms like pronouns and proper names, all other lexical items are classified as predicates with verbal, nominal or adjectival specifications (Rauh 2010). Verbal predicates (V) fulfill the prototypical predicative functions, nominal predicates (N) prototypically function as heads of terms and adjectival predicates (A) are primarily used in attributive functions. While this seems logical with respect to N and V, the A category is arguably not applicable to all languages. However, Dik argues that some languages might use the same forms to express two functions, such as V and A in Bahasa Indonesia, specifying the corresponding predicates as VA (Dik 1997:195). Applying this classification to the ISL data, the syntactic category of referential phrases is clearly associated with N, while modifier

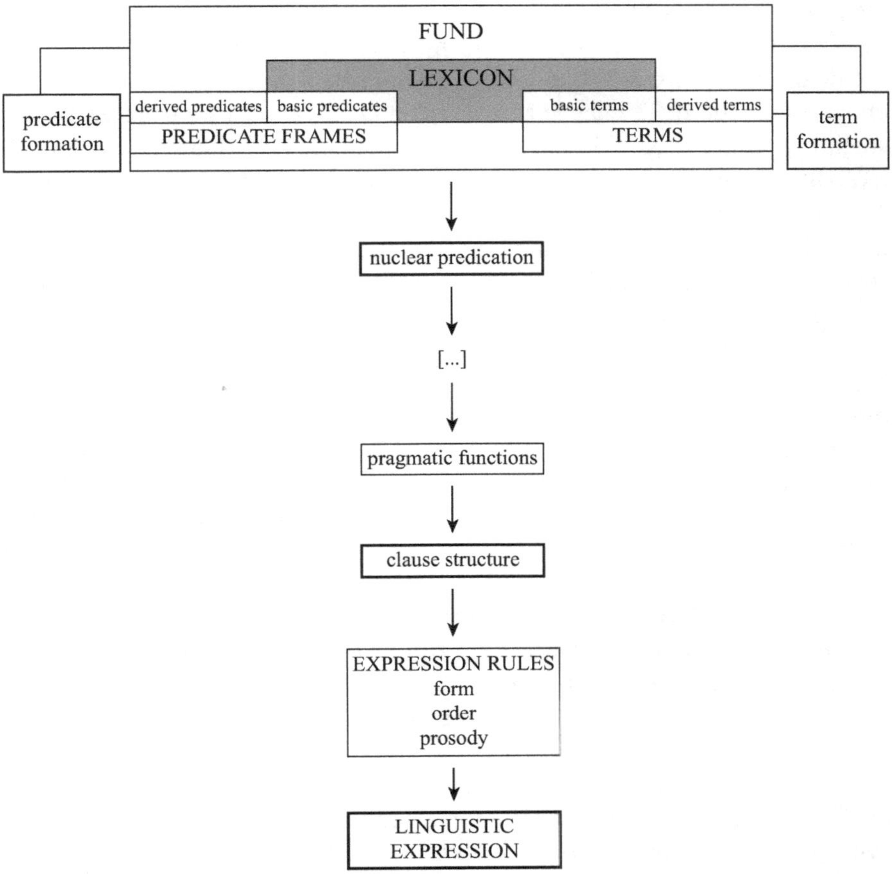

Figure 6.9 Dik's model of functional grammar (modified)

phrases are linked to A. Concerning V, it can be filled by two different forms, either bare or (full) predicates.[92] This split of the V category in ISL is purely based on form and distribution, the basic function of both predicate categories is that of predication though.

In order to determine the structure of nuclear predications, predicates are represented as predicate frames of the structure (Dik 1997:59):

give [V] $(x_1: \langle anim \rangle (x_1))_{Ag} (x_2)_{Go} (x_3: \langle anim \rangle (x_3))_{Rec}$

This represents the valency structure of a V like *give*, with three arguments (x_1, x_2, x_3) and their semantic functions as Agent, Goal and Recipient. Nuclear predications are then formed by inserting basic or derived terms into argument positions like x_1: (x_1: *John* [N] $(x_1))_{Ag}$. Derived terms are formed by term-derivation rules which will however not be discussed here.[93] ISL predicate frames for a V like $_{P1}$GIVE$_{P2}$ would be similar to the one depicted above, with the difference that x_1 (Ag) and x_3 (Rec) would be expressed spatially, while x_2 would constitute a movement. The citation form of a V like GIVE would therefore be similar to a spoken language item like *give*. A major difference to the spoken language predication would be that a V like ISL GIVE would feature another semantic role, namely the Theme represented by a classifier. This would be an essential part of the predicate frame, as opposed to spoken language elements.

Before the level of pragmatic function that is depicted in figure 6.9, several other layers of rules and operators are applied to the nuclear predication. They are not central for situating the ISL data in the grammatical model and are consequently not commented on here. The pragmatic functions depicted in the above figure are that of Topic and Focus and finally derive clause structure. Mouth actions are central in this regard as they can function as one of the markers of focus, for instance (Boyes Braem 2001).

In order to form linguistic expressions, expression rules have to be applied to the clause structure (cf. figure 6.9). These consist of formal expression rules, order-determining expression rules and prosodic rules. Of these, only the first two are important for the study of PoS and will be discussed here.

Formal expression rules correspond to morphological inflection rules or the formal parameter mentioned in chapter 6.1. They might also introduce syntactically autonomous forms such as adpositions, for instance, that fulfill similar functions to inflections (Rauh 2010). This function is often fulfilled by movement or spatial specifications in sign languages, such as a repetition of the movement parameter of a noun in ISL hence representing the inflectional ending for the plural or the movement path of a verb like ‘give’ thus representing the inflection for person.

Placement or order-determining expression rules map constituents of the clause structure to their final positions in the sentence structure. These rules are consequently comparable to the syntactic parameter mentioned in chapter 6.2. These ordering patterns are accounted for by certain ordering principles whose choice is functionally determined. Two of these principles are especially important for sign languages and the syntactic structures frequently found in them (Dik 1997:399):

> (GP_1): *The Principle of Iconic Ordering* […] ordering in one way or another iconically reflects the semantic content of the expression […]

> (GP_7): *The Principle of Pragmatic Highlighting* [...] (New Topic, Given Topic, Completive Focus, Contrastive Focus) are preferably placed in "special positions", including, at least, the clause-initial position

As was mentioned in chapter 2, sign languages are often claimed to be topic prominent languages which means that GP_7 often operates on sign language sentences. As mentioned above, this might coincide with other means of highlighting certain elements, such as mouthings. The importance of iconicity was already discussed at length in several chapters of this book and will not be repeated here. The only syntactic phenomenon that has not been mentioned explicitly in this context is serial verb constructions that have been found to be abundant in sign languages (e.g. Supalla 1990). These constructions are based on the principle of grammatical iconicity (e.g. Aikhenvald 2006) which is thus highly relevant for sign languages.

This short description of functional linguistic theories, Dik's model of functional grammar has clearly situated the results from the analysis of the ISL data presented in chapters 6.2.1 and 6.2.2 in a functional framework. Being concerned with mouth actions in this book, a comment on their placement and functions in this framework seems necessary. Due to their heterogeneous nature, the different types of mouth actions are also situated at different points in the above model.

Concerning mouthings, TYPE 1 (formally and semantically congruent), 3a+b (prepositional verbs and classifiers) and 5 (reduced) mouthings are usually part of basic predicates or terms (in that case of proper names). TYPE 2 (semantically similar but formally different) mouthings are best described as part of the predicate frames as they are not fully part of the basic predicate or term as it occurs in the lexicon. TYPE 4 (inflected English) mouthings are actually formational expression rules that operate on the clause structure. Thus, they function as inflections. TYPE 6a (adding a nuance of meaning) + c mouthings contribute to the pragmatic functions of a clause, as was mentioned above. TYPE 6b (spread) mouthings are at the interface of formational and placement expression rules as they are concerned with the marking of terms on the one hand and syntactical distribution on the other.

With respect to mouth gestures, there is a dichotomous distinction between either forming part of basic predicates (semantically empty mouth gestures) or constituting basic predicates themselves (enacting and adverbial mouth gestures).

As was shown here, similar to their heterogeneous nature, mouth actions also fulfill a variety of different functions when mapped onto a functional grammatical framework.

Chapter 7
Conclusion

The point of departure for the current study was several research questions. Firstly, this book investigated whether different kinds of mouth actions that have been generally distinguished in sign linguistic literature can be found in ISL. Secondly, I elaborated on the question whether these different kinds of mouth actions are used systematically while in a second step trying to determine their respective functions. Finally, the correlation of different kinds of mouth actions with certain sociolinguistic (gender, age) and linguistic (word class) factors was discussed.

One of the results of this investigation is that the different kinds of mouth actions that have been postulated in the literature can also be distinguished for ISL. Apart from the traditional dichotomy of mouth gestures and mouthings that is described in the literature, a more fine-grained typology of mouthings and mouth gestures could be achieved. With respect to mouthings, six distinct types with different functions on the linguistic as well as metalinguistic level, could be established. At first glance, the findings from the SOI seem to support the general claim that mouthings tend to be semantically redundant. However, I suggest that mouthings are rather semantically congruent with a certain manual sign. This acknowledges the fact that all mouthings fulfill certain functions that are relevant for the linguistic setup of a sign or the discourse as a whole. Mouthings are thus in some cases integral parts of signs and might in other cases function as metalinguistic remarks in narratives or as prosodic linkers, especially between pronouns/indeces and content signs. This supports Boyes Braem (2001) and Bank et al.'s (2011) claims that for some signs, mouthings are firmly established parts of the respective signs.[94] Bank and colleagues also suggest that some NGT mouthings might be the result of congruent lexicalization. This could not be proven however, as they only looked at signs in isolation. The current study on ISL sustains the statement that mouthings might fulfill functions that exceed purely lexical purposes and are related to narrative and/or prosodic structure. However, the amount of variation found among mouthings for one sign in ISL (and other sign languages such as NGT) hints at the fact that in many cases mouthings are not lexically determined. This is further substantiated by the rarity of homonyms distinguished by mouthings in ISL and is also in line with Ebbinghaus and Heßmann (2001) who, despite acknowledging the importance for mouthings and the oral-aural modality for sign language structures, do not claim lexical determinacy of mouthings (cf. chapter 3.2.3).

Concerning mouth gestures, it was found that there are three distinct types, namely semantically empty, adverbial and enacting mouth gestures. The latter two types are often iconic in nature and constitute a lexical class of its own, as was shown in chapter 6.2.4. Having established these different types of mouth actions and their functions, it became clear that they are used systematically in order to fulfill said functions. Consequently, they are equally functionally important for the linguistic structure of ISL, which is in line with earlier findings for other sign languages (cf. chapter 3.2.1). Moreover, it became evident that the variation between mouthings and mouth gestures used with the same manual sign that has been reported for NGT for the first time (Bank et al. 2011), can also be observed in ISL. This was shown in chapter 6.2.3 and will be taken up again below.

In the sociolinguistic part of the analysis, the influence of the factors gender and age, of which gender has been extensively researched for ISL, was investigated. While differences concerning both factors individually were clearly visible, one of the main results of this analysis was the interrelation of both factors. A huge discrepancy between the mouth action behaviour of men and women was visible in that men generally use less mouthings than women. This fact could be related to the differences in education and especially the introduction of the oral education method to the Cabra deaf schools at different points in time. Signers of the oldest age group (age group 3) also used less mouthings than signers of the youngest age group (age group 1). This development towards an increased use of English mouthings in present day ISL could also be traced back to the differences in education just mentioned. Further, a higher degree of ISL/English bilingualism in signers which might ultimately further a more frequent use of mouthings seems to be another explanation. Based on Mohr (2012), it was suggested that a monolingual setting in the traditional sense does not exist for deaf people and that we need to rethink and reformulate sociolinguistic frameworks dealing with language contact and bilingualism accordingly. Finally, the increased use of mouthings along with their specific functions in younger generations hints at a firm integration of these items into the linguistic system of ISL. Especially this development over time suggests that a language change has taken place in ISL. However, this language change does by no means support Keller's hypothesis that the frequency and importance of mouthings reduces over time as mentioned in chapter 3.2.3. The data clearly refute his claim that mouthings will eventually fall out of use, in describing the opposite development: an increase in the frequency and importance of mouthings in ISL.

The second part of the investigation was concerned with the question of the correlation between mouth actions and word classes or morphological complexity. In a first step, the word classes of ISL, distinguishing syntactic categories and lexical classes were established. These were found by applying a combination of morphological, morphosyntactic and distributional criteria. Semantic and ontological features were only minor in this respect, and applied in a last step in order to establish possible semantic cores for each lexical class. ISL was found to have four distinct syntactic categories and five lexical classes which do not coincide. Consequently, it was found to be a TYPE B language according to Sasse's (1993a) classification.

Especially the lexical class of verbs proved interesting, as the traditional tripartite division of sign language verbs according to Padden (1988) was found to be inapplicable to the ISL data. In line with earlier studies on ISL, a different distinction into two kinds of verbs, namely full verbs and aktionsart verbs, was established. Finally, the claim that mouth actions might serve as a modality-specific tool for word class recognition in sign languages was followed up on. It was found that mouth actions do not seem to be a useful tool for PoS distinction in ISL as only predicates and the lexical class of verbs can be singled out from the other lexical classes by correlation with different kinds of mouth actions.[95] However, the sub-categorization of the verb class is supported by the analysis of mouth actions. It was observed that a high co-occurrence with mouth gestures reflects a high morphological complexity of a sign whereas a frequent co-occurrence with mouthings mirrors the simpler morphological structure of the respective sign.

Finally, the results from the PoS analysis of the ISL data were situated within the framework of functional linguistic theories and Dik's (1989) model of functional grammar. It turned out that the model is largely applicable to the ISL data, the only difference being that V predications show a split into bare and (full) predicates in ISL which seems to be modality-dependent and holds true for other sign languages as well. In conclusion, the different types of mouth actions were mapped onto the grammatical model proposed by Dik. Reflecting their heterogeneous nature, the different types of mouth actions were also situated at different places of the model, either as basic terms and predicates, predicate frames, pragmatic functions or formal expression rules.

In conclusion, from a functional linguistic point of view, mouth actions are a linguistically important, indispensable part of ISL that fulfills predetermined linguistic and metalinguistic functions. These functions usually cannot be fulfilled by other linguistic means. While this has been undisputed for mouth gestures for a while, it is especially important with respect to mouthings. Contrary to claims that they are not part of the linguistic system of a sign language and could hence be dispensed with (cf. e.g. Hohenberger & Happ 2001), they have been shown to be fully integrated linguistic material of ISL that is essential for the functioning of the linguistic system as a whole. Referring to the "continuum of mouthings as outcomes of code-blending on the one and fully lexicalized items of a sign language on the other end" mentioned by Bank et al. (2011:251), this book positions mouthings towards the lexicalised end of the scale. This does not deny their origin as a language contact phenomenon and the importance of contact between ISL and spoken English for the development of the phenomenon. However, the oral-aural modality has always been available to signers to a certain extent and played a significant role due to the social development of the majority of deaf children in hearing families. The introduction of oralism and the resulting heightened level of sign and spoken language contact only functioned as an enforcing factor. Linguistic change in this context rather refers to the natural evolution of all languages that can be observed more closely in the case of sign languages as young languages. Gaining more and more diverse functions, the final results of the development that started in the 1940s/50s with the introduction of oralism to the Cabra schools remain to be seen and will be an exciting topic of research for future studies.

Appendix A – Complete list of signs and fingerspellings with mouthings[96]

	Sign	Mouthing
A	ABLE	notable
	AGE	age
	AGO	ago
	ALL+lo	that'sall
	a.m.y.	amy
	AOIFE (signname)	aoife
	APARTMENT	apartment
	ART	art
	ASK	ask
	a.s.k.	ask
	ASK+fr	ask
	ASK+sl	ask
	AUDIENCE	crowd
B	BABY	baby
	BACK	attheback
	b.a.c.k.	back
	BACK-GARDEN	backgarden
	BAD	bad
	b.a.i.l.e.y.	baileys
	BALL	ball
	b.a.l.l.y.f.e.r.m.o.n.t.	ballyfermont
	BANANA-BOAT	bananaboat
	b.a.g.k.o.k.	bangkok
	b.a.r.b.a.r.a.	barbara
	BASKETBALL	bounceball
	BEAUTIFUL	beautiful
	BED	bed
	BELIEVE	can't
	BELIEVE	then
	BEST	best
	BETTER	betterthanus
	BETTER	mean
	b.i.	beige
	BICYCLE	ladder

	BICYCLE	bicycle
	BICYCLE	bike
	BIG	big
	BIG	massive
	BLACK	blackrock
	BOOB-HANGING-OUT	boobhangout
	BOOKED	booked
	BORING	boring
	b.o.o.t.e.r.s.t.o.w.n.	booterstown
	BOTH	both
	BOY	bo
	BOY	boy
	BOY	boys
	BOYS	boys
	BREAK	broke
	BREAK	carbroke
	BREAK	goaway
	BREAK	in
	BRILLIANT	brilliant
	BRING	brought
	BROTHER	brother
	BROWN	brown-thomas
	BUS-CONDUCTOR	conductor
	BUS-CONDUCTOR	whatever
	BUSINESS	business
	BUSY	busy
	BUY	bought
	BUY	buy
	BUY	buybuybuy
	BUY	buytwo
	BUY	old
C	CALL	call
	CALM-DOWN	relax
	CAN	can
	CAN	no
	CAN+++	can
	CAN'T-HEAR	can't
	CAN'T-HEAR	can'thear
	CAR	car

CAR	thatcar
c.a.r.	car
CAR-PARK	carpark
CELEBRATION	celebrate
CHAIR	chair
c.h.a.i.r.	chair
c.h.e.c.k.	check
c.h.i.a.n.g.m.a.i.	chiangmai
CHILD	children
COME	come
COME	mainstreamschool
COME-BACK	back
COME-BACK	come
COME-BACK	goback
COME-DOWN	come
COME-HERE	comehere
COME-OVER	back
COME-OVER	join
COME-TOGETHER	team
COMFORTABLE	comfortable
c.o.n.d.u.c.t.o.r.	conductors
CONTINUE	continue
CONTINUE+	continue
COUNTRY++	country
COURSE	course
COURT	court
c.r.e.t.e.	crete
CROSS	cross
c.r.u.m.l.i.n.	crumlin
CUP-OF-TEA	cappuccino
2XCL-VEYEGAZE-MEET	bothsarah-jane
CL-INDEXTHUMB EXTENDED+f	celebrate
c+GO-TO+sl	go
sr+COME-BACK+sl	back
sl+COME-TO+c	comewithme
CL-ISL-L+me	me
CL-ISL-LBENT+me	ladder
CL-INDEX+2hWITH	with
CL-ISL-L+me	whatever

	CL-ISL-LBENT+me	ignore
	CL-INDEXTHUMB EXTENDED+me	sign
	CL-INDEXPERSON+sr	conductor
	CL-ISL-LBENT+me	me
D	d.	dunlaoghaire
	DAUGHTER	daughter
	DAY	day
	DEAD	dead
	DEAF	deaf
	DEAF	ffffffourdeaf
	DEAF	see
	d.e.a.f.	deaf
	DEFEND	defend
	DESCRIBE	describe
	DESCRIBE	explain
	DIFFERENT	different
	DIFFERENT	fsh
	DIFFERENT++	different
	DIFFERENT++	differentdifferentnot
	DISAPPOINT	disappointed
	DO	dowhat
	DO	two
	d.o.g.	dog
	DOG-COMES-BACK	backwon’t
	DONE	finish
	DON’T-KNOW	don’tknow
	DON’T-KNOW	don’tknowwhat
	DRAMA	drama
	DRAW	draw
	DRINK	drink
	DRIVE	drive
	DRIVE	have
	DRIVE+fr	drive
	DRIVE-ME-MAD	drivememad
	DRUNK	drunk
E	EAMON-HAYES(signname)	eamon
	EAMON-HAYES(signname)	eamon-hayes

	EAMON-HAYES(signname)	eamoneamon
	EAMON-HAYES(signname)	toeamon's
	EAT	eat
	EMPATHY	empathy
	EMPTY	empty
	END	endup
	END-UP-DRUNK	enddog
	ENGINE	engine
	ENGINE	turnonthere
	ENJOY	enjoy
	ENGLAND	england
	ENTER	house
	ENOUGH	enough
	EURO	euro
	EURO	threeeuro
	EVENING	evening
	EXCITED	excited
	EXPECT	expect
	EXPENSIVE	that'sexpensive
	EXPERIENCE	experience
	EXPLAIN	explain
	EXPLAIN++	explain
F	FALL	ballfell
	FALL-DOWN	land
	FALSE	fake
	FAMILY	family
	f.e.b.	february
	FEEL	feel
	FINAL	final
	FIND	find
	FIND	found
	FINISH	finish
	FINISH	finished
	FINISH	fsh
	FIX	repairs
	FIX	different
	FLUORESCENT-LIGHT	lantern
	FLUORESCENT-LIGHTS-FLICKING-ON	light

	FOLLOW	follow
	FOLLOW	forward
	FOOL	fool
	f.o.o.l.	fool
	FORM	form
	FORWARD	forward
	FOUND	found
	FRIEND	friend
	FRIEND	fr
	FRIEND	myfriend
	FRIEND	withfriend
	FULL	full
	FUNNY	fun
	FUNNY	funny
G	GAME	game
	GANG	gang
	GARDEN	garden
	GARAGE	garage
	g.a.r.a.g.e.	garage
	GET	get
	GET-ALL-TOGETHER	get
	GIRL	girl
	GIVE	givejust
	GIVE-TO-ME	giveme
	g.o.	goahead
	GO	goon
	GO-BACK	back
	GO-BACK	go
	GO-IN	go
	GO-OFF	go
	g.o.-o.n.	show
	GO-OVER	go
	GO-TO	go
	GO-TO	goto
	GOOD	good
	GREAT	great
	GREAT	was
	GREECE	greece
	GUINESS	guiness

H	HALF	half
	HALF++	halfhalfhalf
	HAND	hand
	HANDBAG	bag
	HAPPY	happy
	HAPPY	nothappy
	HAPPY++	happy
	HAROLD'S	harold's
	HAVE	different
	HAVE	have
	HAVE	sleep
	HAVE	yourself
	h.a.v.e.	have
	HEAD	head
	h.e.a.d.	head
	HEAD	goahead
	HEAR	hears
	HEARING	hearing
	HEART-BROKEN	heart-broken
	HEAT	heat
	HELP	help
	HELP++	help
	HIM	him
	h.i.r.e.	hire
	HOLD	hold
	HOLD-OBJECT-AND-HANDBAG	bagfuckshit
	HOLD-OBJECT-AND-HANDBAG	two
	HOLIDAY	holidays
	HOME	forhome
	HOME	home
	HOME	ho
	HOME+sl	home
	HOPE	hope
	HOT	hot
	HOUSE	house
	h.o.u.s.e.	house
	HOW	how
	HURRY	quick

	HUSBAND	husb
	HUSBAND	myhusband
I	IDENTITY	identity
	IDS	ids
	IGNORE	ignore
	2xCL-INDEX+b+sr	bring
	INDEX+f	Ah!
	INDEX+f	blackrock
	INDEX+f	go
	INDEX+f	gone
	CL-INDEX+f	oh
	INDEX+f	tellmy
	INDEX+f	thankyou
	INDEX+f	this
	INDEX+f	wants
	INDEX+f	with
	INDEX+f	wrong
	INDEX+f	you
	INDEX+f,down	have
	INDEX+f,hi	blackrock
	CL-INDEX+f+hi	that
	INDEX+f,lo	engine
	INDEX+fl,lo	before
	INDEX+fl,lo	that
	INDEX+fl	because
	INDEX+fl	funny
	INDEX+fl	outside
	INDEX+fl	them
	INDEX+fl	think
	INDEX+fl	work
	INDEX+fr	ask
	INDEX+fr	he
	INDEX+fr	it
	INDEX+fr	out
	INDEX+fr	that
	INDEX+fr	willing
	INDEX+fr	friend
	INDEX+fr	won'tmovehethink
	INDEX+fr,hi	hear

INDEX+fr,hi	there
INDEX+fr,hi	to
INDEX+fr,lo	he
INDEX+fr,lo	her
INDEX+fr,lo	talking
INDEX+hi,fr	Ireland
INDEX+me	ago
INDEX+me	ask
INDEX+me	back
INDEX+me	besideme
INDEX+me	buybuybuy
INDEX+me	chair
INDEX+me	comewithme
INDEX+me	first
INDEX+me	forme
INDEX+me	fumes
INDEX+me	go
INDEX+me	have
INDEX+me	haveto
INDEX+me	help
INDEX+me	hold
INDEX+me	I
INDEX+me	it
INDEX+me	jump
INDEX+me	ladder
INDEX+me	lead
INDEX+me	leave
INDEX+me	leftkeep
INDEX+me	look
INDEX+me	me
CL-INDEX+me	me
INDEX+me	my
INDEX+me	noharmnoharm
INDEX+me	not
INDEX+me	now
INDEX+me	oh
INDEX+me	photograph
INDEX+me	points
INDEX+me	realise
INDEX+me	saint

INDEX+me	saturday
INDEX+me	thailand
INDEX+me	to
INDEX+me	tomorrow
INDEX+me	tuesday
INDEX+me	wait
INDEX+me	want
INDEX+me	we
INDEX+me	went
INDEX+me	wife
INDEX+me	will
INDEX+me	willnot
INDEX+me	with
INDEX+me	wasgreat
INDEX-RIGHTSIDE	drama
INDEX+sl	boy
INDEX+sl	can
INDEX+sl	garage
INDEX+sl	know
INDEX+sl	you
INDEX+sl+hi	son
INDEX+sr	gooffffffff
INDEX+sr	his
INDEX+sr	join
INDEX+sr	let
INDEX+sr	mean
INDEX+sr	oh!
INDEX+sr	see
INDEX+sr	showus
INDEX+sr	think
INDEX+sr	week
INDEX+sr	whatdo
INDEX+sr,lo	after
INDEX+sr,lo	him
INDEX+sr,lo	that'sexpensive
INDEX+we	betterthanus
INDICATOR-RISES-ON-GAUGE	level
INFORMATION	information
INTEREST	interesting

	CL-ISL-LBENT+me	sorry
	IRELAND	ireland
	IT	it
	IT	took
J	JOB	job
	JOB	work
	j.o.b.	job
	JOIN	seconds
	JOSEPH	joseph
	JUMP++	jumpjump
	JUMP-OVER-OBJECT	jump
K	KEEN	formy
	KEEP	keep
	KNEEL	kneeldown
	KNOW	all
	KNOW	brown-thomas
	KNOW	didn't
	KNOW	hope
	KNOW	know
L	LADDER	ladder
	LADDER	ladderladder
	LANGUAGE	l-
	LAST	last
	LEAD	lead
	l.e.a.k.	check
	LEAK	in
	LEAK++	leak
	LEARN	learn
	LEARN++	learning
	LEAVE	day
	LEAVE	left
	LEAVE	toleave
	LEAVE	whatever
	LEAVE-IT	leave
	LECTURE	lecture
	LEFT	left
	LET	let

	LIFE	life
	LIFT	lift
	LIFT-OFF	off
	LIGHT	lantern
	LIKE	like
	LIKE	love
	LIVE	live
	LOOK	look
	LOOK	lookright
	LOOK-FOR	look
	LOOK-FORWARD	forward
	LOOK-UP	look
	LONG	long
	LOST	lost
	LOT	alot
	LOT	load
	LOVE	love
	LUCKY	lucky
M	MAINSTREAM-SCHOOL	mainstreamschool
	MAKE	fool
	MAKE	makeup
	MAKE	makesure
	MAN	man
	MAN	my
	MARY	mary's
	m.a.t.	mat
	MATCH	match
	MEAN	mean
	MEAN	will
	m.e.d.o.w.	meadow
	MEET-PERSON	meetmeetmeet
	MEMORY	memory
	MISS	miss
	MIX	happy
	MONDAY	Monday
	MONEY	money
	MONTH	month
	MONTH	two
	MONTHS	months

	MORE	more
	MORNING	inthemorning
	MORNING	morning
	MOTHER	mother
	MOTORBIKE	scooter
	MOTORBIKE	scooting
	MOVE-MOTORBIKE	move
	MY	my
N	NAME	name
	n.b.a.	nba
	n.e.a.r.	nearly
	NEED	need
	NEW	new
	NEXT	next
	n.e.x.t.	nextweek
	NICE	nice
	NIGHT	night
	n.i.g.h.t.	night
	n.i.s.s.a.n.	nissan
	NORMAL	normal
	NORTH-IRELAND	northireland
	NOTHING	nothing
O	OFFICE	office
	OKAY	fine
	OKAY	goahead
	OKAY	ok
	OKAY	willbeokay
	OLD	older
	ONLY	only
	OTHER	other
	OVER	over
	OVER-NIGHT-TRAIN	overnighttrain
	OWN	own
P	PACKING-UP	pack
	PAPER	paper
	PART	p-
	p.a.r.t.	part

	PERCENT	fifitypercent
	PERCENT	percent
	PERFECT	fabulous
	PERFECT	great
	PERFECT	perfect
	PERSON	know
	PHOTOGRAPH	photograph
	PHOTOGRAPH	photos
	PLATE	plate
	PLAY	play
	p.l.u.g.s.	plugs
	POINT	point
	POINT	points
	POSSESSIVE+fr	friend
	POSSESSIVE+fr	his
	POSSESSIVE+sl	he
	POUR-INTO-TANK	fill
	PRACTISE	pra-pra
	PREPARE	prepare
	p.r.i.m.a.	prima
	PROBLEM	problem
	PUB	pub
	p.u.m.p.	pump
	PUT	put
	PUT-SMALL-OBJECT-IN-ENGINE	putin
R	r.d.s.	rds
	READ-PAPER	read
	READY	ready
	REAL	really
	REALISE	realise
	REDUCE	cheap
	REDUCE	fiftypercent
	REDUCE	lucky
	REMEMBER	remember
	REMOVE-PARTS-OF-ENGINE	off
	REMOVE-PARTS-OF-ENGINE++	offoff

	REMOVE-PARTS-OF-ENGINE+++	offoffoff
	REMOVE-PARTS-OF-ENGINE+++++	offoffoffoffoff
	REPEAT++	repeatrepeat
	REST	rest
	RIGHT	lookright
	RIGHT	right
	RIGHT	rightshoes
	ROB	rob
	r.o.w.	row
	RUN	run
S	SAINT	saint
	SAME	same
	SAME	samesamesame
	SAORISE(signname)	saorise
	SARAH-JANE(signname)	sarah-jane
	SATURDAY	saturday
	SAY	dunlaoghaire
	SAY	eamon-hayes
	SAY	said
	SAY	will
	SCORE-IN-BASKETBALLNET	scored
	SCOTLAND	scotland
	SCHOOL	inschool
	SCHOOL	school
	SEANEOGHAN(signname)	seaneoghan
	SEATS	seats
	SECOND	minute
	SEE	blackrock
	SEE	bought
	SEE	eamon
	SEE	have
	SEE	hear
	SEE	photos
	SEE	saw
	SEE	see
	SEE	wantsee

SEE	willsee
SEE-BEFORE	feel
SELF	own
SELF	self
SELF	yourself
s.e.m.i.	semi
SEMI-FINAL	semi-final
SHAPE-OF-CHAIR-HANDLES	chairfor
SHAPE-OF-SHELL	I
SHELL	shellllll
SHOES	forshoes
SHOES	shoes
SHOP	shop
s.h.o.p.	shop
SHOPPING	shop
SHORTS	shorts
SHOULD	should
SHOVEL	xdgp
SHOW	show
s.h.o.w.	showus
SICK	sick
SIGN	sign
SIGNING	goon
SIGNING	sign
SIT	sit
SLEEP	sleep
SMALL	small
SMELL	smell
SMELL-RISE-UP	smell
SON	son
SORRY	sorry
START	start
s.t.a.y.	greece
STOP	stop
STORY	continue
STORY	onestory
STORY	story
STRIPES-ON-TOP-OF-SHOES	brownbeige

	STRONG	strong
	STUPID	stupid
	SUMMERCAMP	summercamp
	s.u.n.	jump
	SUN	sun
	SUNDAY	sunday
	SUN-SHINING	sun
	SURE	sure
	SWEET	sweet
T	TAKE	took
	TALK	talking
	TALK-TO-EACH-OTHER	chatchat
	t.a.l.l.a.g.h.t.	tallaght
	TANK-FILLS-UP	fillup
	TEAM	team
	TELL	tell
	TELL+fl	told
	TELL+fr	tell
	THAILAND	thailand
	THANK	thankyou
	THERE	believe
	THERE	turnonthere
	THING	everything
	THING	something
	THINK	bighead
	THINK	see
	THINK	think
	t.h.i.n.k.	think
	THINK	thought
	THINK	won'tmovehethink
	THIS	this
	THOMAS-O'CALLAGHAN	thomas
	THOMAS-OCALLAGHAN	true
	THOUGHT	thought
	THROW-AWAY	saw
	THROW-BALL-UP	throw
	THROW-OUT	throw
	TOGETHER	comewithme
	TOUCH	feel

	TIME	first
	TIME	sametime
	TIME	time
	TIME++	timetimetime
	TIRED	tired
	TIRED	inthemorning
	TRAINING	train
	TRUE	true
	TRY	try
	TRY	tryto
	TUESDAY	tuesday
	TURN-KEY-OFF	gooffff
	TURN-KEY-ON	switch
	TURN-KEY-ON	tu-
	TV+	tv
U	UK	uk
	UNA	una
	UNDERSTAND	understand
	UNDERSTAND	understandbut
	US	showus
V	VEHICLE-MOVE	won'tmovehethink
	VIDEO	film
W	WAIT	wait
	WAKE-UP	wake
	WALES	wales
	WALL	thewall
	WALK	forwalk
	WALK	walk
	WALK+++++++++	walkwalkwalkwalkwalkwalk
	WALK-AROUND	see
	WALK-AROUND+sl	check
	WALKING	willnot
	WALKING-STICK	stick
	WANT	wa-
	WANT	want
	WANT	wants
	WASTE	waste

	WAS	was
	WATCH	clock
	WATCH	watch
	WATER	water
	WAY	way
	WEAVED	twistortweed
	WEDNESDAY	Wednesday
	WEEK	nextweek
	WEEK	week
	w.e.l.l.	well
	WENT-OVER	go
	w.e.x.f.o.r.d.	wexford
	WHAT	what's
	WHISTLE	whistle
	WHO	who
	WIFE	wife
	WILL++	will
	WILL-BE	willbeokay
	WILL-NOT	will
	WILL-NOT	willnot
	WILL-NOT	won'tmovehethink
	WILLING	willing
	WIN	towin
	WIN	win
	WIN	won
	WINDOW	window
	w.o.o.d.	wood
	WON'T	won't
	WORK	no
	WORLD	world
	WORRY	worry
	w.r.o.n.g.	wrong
Y	YEAR	year
	YEAR	years
	y.e.a.r.	ten
	YEARS	foryears
	YOUNG	young
	YOUR	your

Appendix B – Contexts for examples (glossed with mouthings)

Contexts are given for approximately 5 seconds before and 5 seconds after the instance given in the example. The first line indicates the mouthing, the second the gloss.[97] Finally, a rough translation is provided.

Example 1

chapter 4 (p. 70): index+me index+fl index+me 'sure just leave it for now'
Taken from Fergus D., 00:45.

closed, stretched_______ "fill up"______
Index-me POUR-INTO-TANK TANK-FILLS-UP SCREW-CAP-ON

closed, stretched down_____________ open__ "continue"
'what's the problem?' index-me DRIVE WATER CONTINUE PROBLEM

closed, stretched down____ "oh!"_______________
Index-me index-fl index-me 'sure just leave it for now'

"see" "my"___"friend" "have" closed, stretched down "car"
Index-me SEE index-me FRIEND HAVE index-fr KNOW^SKILL ABOUT CAR

"repairs"
FIX DIFFER POSSESSIVE-fr

"ask"______
index-me ASK index-lo 'what's the problem?'

'I poured [water] into the tank, it filled up and I screwed the cap on. What was the problem? I drove [on] but still had the water problem. I thought 'just leave it for now'. I saw my friend [who] has several cars and knows about car repairs. I asked him 'what's the problem, what's wrong?'.'

Example 2

chapter 4 (p. 70): OKAY 'let's go then', 'sauntering over', thumbs up
Taken from Laurence, 01:09

"me"___ "both" open, left lower corner down
Index-me BOTH index-me 'boys look at each other' index-sl index-me

WHAT-TO-DO

"one" wrinkled nose, open, left corner up
index-sl ONE DEAF SAY CURIOUS index-f-hi

open, wrinkled nose stretched down, closed, forward open, wrinkled nose, left corner up
OKAY 'let's go then' 'sauntering over' thumbs up

forward, stretched down, closed closed, round, stretched down
BOY 'shows off bike'

closed, stretched down closed, forward, stretched down "nice" closed, forward,
MOTORBIKE index-fr SEE NICE 'extent of

stretched down open, left corner up
motorbike' thumbs up 'that's that'

'[The group of boys] looked at the deaf guy. [The deaf guy said] 'come over here, look at the bike.' [The group of boys said] 'come over here with the motorbike.' Me and my friend we both looked at each other and wondered what to do. Then one deaf guy said 'this is a curious deaf boy.' [The group of boys said] 'let's go then' and sauntered over. They motioned a thumbs-up. The deaf guy showed off his motorbike. The deaf guy said 'look at this very nice motorbike.'

Example 3

chapter 4 (p.70): 'all done'
Taken from Kevin, 02:39[98]

open, stretched
STORM-OFF

open, round forward open, round, jaw low labiodental, low closed, stretched open
MOTHER ACT-MAD-WITH-FIST

"waste" "time"
WASTE MY TIME

wrinkled nose, labiodental low "fool" wrinkled nose, labiodental low
index-sl MAKE FOOL index-sl FOR

wrinkled nose, stretched, jaw low labiodental low "for" "fool"___
NOT index-sl index-me FOOL FOR MAKE FOOL

"me"
index-me

'I stormed off. [My] mother waved her fist madly and said 'you wasted my time'. 'You have made a fool of yourself and a fool of me."

Example 4

chapter 4 (p. 78): SHOES POINTED-SHOES EXPENSIVE STRIPES-ON-TOP-OF-SHOES *b.i.
Taken from Marian, 01:43

open, stretched_________ labiodental-low___ "to" "prima" "shop"
index-me 'hold on a sec' index-me SEE WALK-AROUND p.r.i.m.a. SHOP

open, jaw low "shoes" closed, round-ao closed, stretched-ao "brown, beige"

index-me LOOK-AT+sr SHOES POINTED-SHOES EXPENSIVE STRIPES-ON-TOP-OF-SHOES b.i.

OH-DEAR SO-FASHIONABLE POSH

'I said 'hold on a sec.' I saw a Prima shop and walked around it. I looked at [a pair of] shoes, which were expensive and had brown and beige stripes on top. Oh dear, they were so fashionable and posh.'

Example 5a

chapter 4 (p. 79): TEAM COME-TOGETHER
Taken from Caroline, 01:14

"three" "seconds" "left" "throw"_________

THREE JOIN LEFT CL-index thumb extended-c THROW-BALL-UP

"me"___ "hope" "ball"____ "land" "match" "over"

index-me KNOW BALL FALL-DOWN MATCH OVER

"ball" "fell" "hear" "final" "whistle"

FALL SEE FINAL WHISTLE

"team" "run" "jump, jump"

index-me TEAM COME-TOGETHER RUN-IN-ACTION JUMP++

"massive" "celebrate"

BIG CELEBRATION CL-thumb extended-f

"the" "end"

END

"definitely" "one" "best" "memory" "my" "life"

DEFINITELY ONE BEST MEMORY IN LIFE

'Three seconds were left, one [person] threw the ball up. I knew that when the ball fell down, the match would be over. [The ball] fell down, I saw the final whistle. I saw that the team came together, running around and jumping, jumping. It was a massive celebration. That's the end. That is definitely one of the best memories in [my] life.'

Example 5b

chapter 4 (p. 79): KNOW PERSON
Taken from Fergus D., 01:25

"have" "friend" open, stretched wide "life" "wexford"____
HAVE FRIEND index-fr-hi IN LIVE IN w.e.x.f.o.r.d. index-fr-hi

open, forward, stretched wide "repair"_ "know"_____
GOOD INTEREST HAVE FIX DIFFERENT GOOD index-me KNOW PERSON index-me

"went"________ "drive"
WHERE index-me DRIVE DRIVE-THERE-IN-CAR

"ask"______ "him" "problem" "over" "heat"
ENTER index-fr ASK ABOUT index-f-lo PROBLEM OVER HEAT

'[I] had a friend who lived in Wexford. He had a strong interest in repairing different [engines]. I knew where that person lived. I drove to [his place in my car]. I entered and asked him about the problem of overheating.'

Example 6a

chapter 4 (p. 79): STAY GREECE
Taken from Laurence, 0:12

closed, stretched down "near" "ten" "ago"_
TEN NEAR TEN YEAR AGO

“with” “friend” “fffour” “deaf” open, stretched, left corner up “gang”
WITH FRIEND FOUR DEAF PERSON GANG

closed, stretched, forward
TOGETHER-IN-GROUP ‘HANDS UP’

open, left corner up open_____ “greece” “crete”
GO-OFF STAY STAY GREECE c.r.e.t.e. ‘that’s that’

“two” wrinkled nose, open wrinkled nose, closed, labiodental-low “pub”
TWO MONTH ‘hands-up’ EVERY NIGHT DIFFERENT PUB

‘That was about ten years ago. I went with four deaf friends who were in a gang together, ehm… We went off and stayed in, in Greece. That’s that. For two months, ehm, we spent every night at a different pub.’

Example 6b

chapter 4 (p. 79): ENTER HOUSE
Taken from Fergus D., 03:23

open___ “sleep”
index-me SLEEP

closed, bilabial, tense_____________________
index-fr IGNORE CONTINUE ENDURE FIX-UP

open, teeth clenched______________________
FIX-UP-ALL-PARTS-OF-ENGINE ‘such a big job’

“time, time”
TIME+++

open____ “house”______
‘taking that long?’ index-me ‘leave it’ index-me ‘hands up’ ENTER HOUSE

“have”_______ “house”__ “sleep”___ “chair”
POSSESSIVE-fr HAVE HOUSE index-fl HAVE SLEEP CHAIR

“chair”_______ closed, sides down________
index-me CHAIR index-me[99] SIT ‘arms folded in sleep’ SLEEP

“three”
ABOUT THREE-O’CLOCK

‘I [wanted to] sleep. My friend ignored me and continued fixing up all parts of the engine. That was such a big job! A lot of time passed. What was taking that long? I thought ‘leave it’ and entered the house. My friend had a house with a sleeping chair in it. I sat down in the chair, folded my arms and slept from about three o’clock [...].’

Example 7a

chapter 4 (p. 77): index-me KEEP
Taken from Caroline, 01:01

“look”__________“to” “sarah-jane” “both”
CL-U-bent CL-V-arc-sl-lo to sr-hi TO SARAH-JANE 2X CL-V EYEGAZE-MEET

“know” “we”___ “won” “continue” closed, stretched “play”
KNOW index-me WIN index-me CONTINUE BASKETBALL PLAY

“five” “seconds” “left”
FIVE JOIN LEFT

“keep”____ “look”_ “look” “crowd”_ open, stretched, teeth clenched
index-me KEEP CL-V SL-HI TO F-HI AUDIENCE CL-U-bent-c CL-V-fr-hi CL-V-sl CL-V-sl-hi[100]

‘[Then] I looked over to Sarah-Jane and our eyes met. We both knew we had won. The game continued. Five seconds were left. I looked at the watch, then at the game; the crowd looked at the watch, then back at the game.’

Example 7b

chapter 4 (p. 80): CHAIR index-me

Taken from Fergus D., 03:26

As the context for this example was already given above (cf. example 6b), it is not provided here again.

Example 8

chapter 4 (p. 82): KEEN FOR-MY GARDEN HOLD-OBJECT-AND-HANDBAG

Taken from Marian, 00:38

“eamon”__ “want” “see” “shelllll”____________
EAMON-HAYES SEE SHELL SHAPE-OF-SHELL

closed, forward__ open, jaw low_______________
index-me ‘so what?’ WALK-FROM-RIGHT-TO-LEFT

________________________ “eamon”_______
index-me GET-ATTENTION-OF index-sr EAMON-HAYES++

“never”____ “before” “but”__ closed, forward “for” “my”__ “garden”
index-fl NEVER BEFORE index-fl-low BUT index-me KEEN FOR-MY GARDEN

“bag”__ “fuck, shit”___________ open, stretched “small” “bag”___
HOLD-OBJECT-AND-HANDBAG index-me SMALL HANDBAG

open, stretched up_________
PUT-THINGS-IN-HANDBAG TAKE-SOME-THINGS-OUT-OF-BAG

DAMN-IT

‘Eamon-Hayes wanted to see the shell and its shape. I said ‘so what?’ and walked from right to left. I [tried] to get Eamon-Hayes’ attention repeatedly. I had never [seen something like this] before but I wanted it for my garden. I held the objects and my handbag [but] I had a small handbag. I put some things in the handbag and took some things out. [I thought] ‘damn it!’.’

Example 9

chapter 4 (p. 83): SIGNING STORY SIGNING
Taken from Sarah-Jane, 00:42

"whatever"______ closed, bilabial____________ closed, stretched up
BUS-CONDUCTOR CL-D-CAME OVER pause, hands clasped CL-V LOOK AT ME-fl-fr gesture, hands folded

closed, stretched up____
CL-V LOOK AT ME-fl-fr CL-V LOOK-fr-fl CL-V LOOK AT ME-fl-fr CL-V LOOK-fr-fl CL-V LOOK AT

___
ME fl-c CL-ISL-L-me cl-v look-f

"whatever"_______ closed, stretched up "continue" "go on" closed, stretched up
LEAVE CL-ISL-L-ME SIGNING STORY SIGNING

"again" tongue 30%
AGAIN CL-INDEX-PERSON-sr-sl CL-INDEX-sr-sl CL-INDEX-PERSON-CIRCLE-hi
open, relaxed___
CL-5-me SIGNING

'The bus conductor came over and looked at me. He looked at me, I looked at him, he looked at me, I looked at him, he looked at me, I looked at him. [Then] he left. I continued signing when again several people came by. I continued signing.'

Example 10

chapter 4 (p. 80): INDICATOR-RISES-ON-GAUGE SURPRISE
Taken from Fergus D., 00:22

"for years" closed, stretched, forward______________
YEARS OVER-A-PERIOD-OF-TIME-TO-NOW DAY DRIVE-AROUND

“until” open, corner up “about” “two” “months” “ago”___ closed, stretched down_
UNTIL RECENTLY ABOUT TWO MONTHS index-me DRIVE index-me WHAT'S-THE-PROBLEM

“hot” open, stretched down__
HOT INDICATOR-RISES-ON-GAUGE SURPRISE WHAT'S-THE-PROBLEM

“have” “check” “water”
index-me DRIVE index-me c.h.e.c.k. WALK-AROUND WATER QUANTITY-EMPTY

‘For years I drove around [in my car every] day until recently, about two months ago, I was driving when I [suddenly] noticed a problem. The [engine] was hot, the indicator rose on the gauge. I was surprised and wondered what the problem was. I walked around the car and checked: the water was empty.’

Example 11

chapter 4 (p. 83): index-fr MAN FRIEND
Taken from Fergus D., 01:04

closed, stretched “leak”__ “maybe” “need” “new” “pump” “in”_ “stop”
index-lo index-sl-lo l.e.a.k.x2 index-f? NEED NEW p.u.m.p. LEAK STOP

open, stretched down “but” “he”___ “my” “friend” “have” “booked”
index-fr BUT index-fr MAN FRIEND index-fr HAVE BOOKED

“all”__ “day” “busy” “cannot” “able” open, stretched wide
KNOW LEAVE BUSY NOT ABLE index-me ‘leave it’

‘The car leaks. It needs a new pump to stop the leak. I looked at [my] friend but I knew that he was very busy and not able to leave. So I thought ‘leave it’.’

Example 12

chapter 4 (p. 84): DEAF TEXT-MESSAGE
Taken from Fergus D., 04:06

open___ "leave"_
index-me 'leave it'

"back"________________ "home"
index-me sr-COME-BACK-sl HOME-sl

"next" "day" "see"_____ closed, forward ao "said" "have" "engine" "from" "other" "car"
NEXT DAY index-sr DEAF TEXT-MESSAGE SAY HAVE ENGINE FROM OTHER?

"same" "engine" "one" "point" "six"
SAME ENGINE ONE POINT SIX

'I thought 'leave it'. I went back home. The next day I had a deaf text message that said [he] had an engine from another car. The same engine 1.06.'

Example 1

chapter 6 (p. 134): BOY SOME FUNNY
Taken from Noeleen, 00:43

"office" open "boring" "same, same, same" closed, stretched "but" open, relaxed___"love"
OFFICE BORING SAME++ BUT index-fl index-me LOVE
"it"
IT

"look" "forward" "school"
LOOK FORWARD SCHOOL

"boys" "some" "funny" open, stretched up "sometimes" open, tense, stretched, teeth forward
BOY SOME FUNNY SOMETIMES CL-5open-hands-palms-up

“drive, me, mad”
DRIVE-ME-MAD

open, stretched “but” “good” “experience”
AND BUT GOOD EXPERIENCE

‘In an office it is boring, [every day] is the same. But I loved [work at the school]. I looked forward to it. Some boys are funny, sometimes they drive me mad. And... but it is a good experience.’

Example 2

chapter 6 (p. 134): EAMON-HAYES HAPPY
Taken from Marian, 00:25

“rds” “after” “this” “stop” “for” “cappuccino”
r.d.s. AFTER index-f STOP FOR CUP-OF-TEA

open, forward ao_______ “relax”____ open, stretched ai “happy”
SIGNING-TO-EACH-OTHER CALM-DOWN EAMON-HAYES HAPPY
“break” “go, away”
BREAK AWAY

“chat, chat”___________ “eamon”______ “good”____
TALK-TO-EACH-OTHER EAMON-HAYES THUMBS-UP

“form” “love” open, forward ao “see” “black, rock”_____
FORM LIKE WALK-AROUND SEE BLACK index-f-hi

‘After this we stopped at R.D.S. for a cappuccino. We signed and relaxed. Eamon-Hayes was happy to get away on a break. We talked to each other and Eamon-Hayes told me he loved this. He walked around [the house] and saw a black rock.’

Example 3

chapter 6 (p. 135): FABULOUS PLATE m.a.t.
Taken from Marian, 01:27

open, forward ao__________ "eamon"_____ open, stretched ai open
index-me CHAT-AND-EATING EAMON-HAYES 'wait a minute' EAMON-HAYES 'scream'

"wait"_______
'wait a minute'

"go"________ "m" "medow"_ "shop" "everything" "half" "fifty" "percent"
index-me WENT-OVER m. me.d.o.w. SHOP THING HALF FIFTY PERCENT

"plate" "mat" "twist" open__________ tongue 10% open__________
FABULOUS PLATE m.a.t. WEAVED FABULOUS BUY++ 'not really' BUT 'hold on a sec'

open_____ "hold"______ bilabial____
index-me CURIOUS HOLD index-fr-arc

'I was chatting and eating, when I said to Eamon-Hayes 'wait a minute'. He was startled but I said 'wait a minute'. I went over to the M... Medow Shop which had everything reduced to half price. There was a fabulous weaved plate mat. I considered buying it but thought 'hold on a sec' and had another curious look around.'

Example 4

chapter 6, (p. 135): DIFFERENT PART COUNTRY++
Taken from Marian, 02:30

jaw low, open____ "bought" "shorts" "cheap"____
sl-WALK-OVER-sr SEE BUY SHORTS REDUCE++

“lucky” open, jaw low “suit” “look” “right” “shop” “cheap”
LUCKY ALWAYS SUIT LOOK RIGHT SHOP REDUCE

“different” “p-“ “country”__ “part” closed, stretched up “do, what”__
DIFFERENT PART COUNTRY++ PART ‘what can you do?’ DO ‘ah well’

closed, stretched up “buy, buy, buy”___________
index-me TAKING-THINGS-OFF-SHELF BUY index-me

“finish” “no, money” “finish”
DONE ‘no money’ DONE

‘I walked over and [suddenly] saw shorts that were much reduced. I was always lucky. I looked right and the shop that had the reduced [items] was in a different part of the country. I thought ‘well, what can you do?’. I took things off the shelves until I was done. I said ‘I don’t have any money anymore.’.’

Example 5

chapter 6 (p. 135): THEY NEED ME BAD –LY
Taken from Fergus M., 02:44

LEAVE c.i.e. NOW c.i.e. WOULD GO-INTO-DEBT c.i.e. WOULD GO-INTO-DEBT gesture

closed, round, lips forward
2XCL-5 palms-up

THEY NEED ME BAD –LY THEY NEED ME BAD –LY

‘If [I] left C.I.E. now, they would go into debt. What can you say? They need me badly. They need me badly.’

Example 6

chapter 6 (p. 135): MOTHER [...] DRINK-TEA –ING TEA
Taken from Peter, 02:01

open, stretched wide, sides up
KISS-EACH-OTHER INDEX-ME HAVE BEFORE 2XNO IDEA WHAT HAPPEN

closed, lips tense, stretched wide
KISS-EACH-OTHER BRING

"mother" "son"________
index-sl MOTHER IN THE KITCHEN DRINK –ING TEA WITH BOY SON index-sl-hi

'We kissed each other and I had no idea what would happen. We kissed each other and went in. The mother was in the kitchen drinking tea with her son.'

Example 7

chapter 6 (p. 136): CONDUCTOR CL-5-palm up
Taken from Sarah-Jane,
As the context for this example was already given above (cf. example 9, chapter 4), it is not provided here again.

Example 8

chapter 6 (p. 136): MEET-PERSON++
Taken from Sean, 00:16

"hearing" "mainstream" "school" open, jaw low
HEARING MAINSTREAM SCHOOL COME w.o.w.

“deaf”__________ “deaf” “world” “strong” open, jaw low “meet, meet, meet”
DEAF ALL-AROUND DEAF WORLD STRONG ALL-AROUND MEET-PERSON++

open, jaw low “first” “l-“
SIGN FIRST LANGUAGE

“happy” “have”_ open “banana, boat”
HAPPY MIX HAVE PAUSE BANANA BOAT

‘The [students] from the hearing mainstream school came over and were very excited. There was deaf culture all around, the deaf world was strong [at the camp], you could meet lots of people all around there. Sign was the first language. Everyone was happy and mixed with people. We had… a banana boat.’

Example 9

chapter 6 (p. 137): index-fr WANT SHOVEL GOOD
Taken from Kevin, 00:56

closed, round, forward open_____
MUST SELF SHOVEL GLOVES ? CLOTHES SELF OWN++ CLOTHES ‘thumbs up’ x2

‘wringing hands’

sl-PERSON-GO-TO-LOCATION-FR TELL FATHER index-fr

“dig, up” “want” “how”
WANT SHOVEL GOOD AND WANT SHOW ME HOW PLACE-SHOVEL-F
RIGHT PLACE-SHOVEL DIG-WITH-SHOVEL

‘I had to provide my own shovel, gloves [?] and clothes I owned myself. Right, [I was well prepared]. I went to my father and told him to show me how to correctly dig with a shovel.’

Example 10

chapter 6 (p. 140): HAVE BANANA BOAT

Taken from Sean, 00:21

As the context for this was already partly given above (cf. example 8, chapter 6), only the 5 seconds preceding the sequence are provided.

"have" open "banana, boat" stretched up "funny"
HAVE (pause) BANANA BOAT RIDING-BOAT FUNNY

"fsh"____ "art" "night" "drama"__________ "game" "plenty" "different"__
DIFFERENT ART NIGHT index-right side DRAMA (pause) GAME PLENTY DIFFERENT++

'We had a banana boat and riding that boat was a lot of fun. We had different art nights and drama [nights]… plenty of different games.'

Example 11

chapter 6 (p. 140): r.d.s. AFTER index+f STOP FOR CUP-OF-TEA

Taken from Marian, 0:20

As the context for this was already partly given above (cf. example 2, chapter 6), only the 5 seconds preceding the sequence are provided.

closed, forward_____ closed, round______________________________________
index-me PACKING-UP KEEN PUTTING-ON-SHORTS PUT-CLOTHES-ON-TOP

____
PACKING-UP WALK-ALONG+++

"rds" "after" "this" "stop" "for" "cappuccino"
r.d.s. AFTER index-f STOP FOR CUP-OF-TEA

'I packed up my things, I was keen to get out, I put [my] shorts on and packed some more things. Then we walked for quite a while. After this we stopped at R.D.S. for a cappuccino.'

Example 12

chapter 6 (p. 140): LAST DAY index-sr CRY++
Taken from Sean, 00:29

“game” “plenty” “different”____ “lecture” open, round, stretched
GAME PLENTY DIFFERENT++ LECTURE (pause) INTERESTING

“home” “last” “day” open, jaw low, tongue 10% “heartbroken”_ open, wrinkled nose
HOME LAST DAY index-sr CRY++ HEART^BROKEN CRY

“miss” “friend” open
MISS FRIEND (pause)

“home” “back”__ “normal” “world”
HOME GO-BACK NORMAL WORLD

‘There were plenty of different games and lectures… [It was] interesting. Before going home, on the last day, people cried a lot, they were heartbroken and would miss their friends… At home it was back to the normal world.’

Example 13

chapter 6 (p. 141): EVERY DAY DIFFERENT++ […] OFFICE […] SAME++
Taken from Noeleen, 00:33

As the context for this was already partly given above (cf. example 1, chapter 6), only the 5 seconds preceding the sequence are provided.

“because” “can” “sign” “same” closed, stretched up_____
BECAUSE CAN SIGN SAME CL-K+LOC-TWO-OF-US

“and, um” “interesting” “every” “day” “different, different”
AND INTEREST EVERY DAY DIFFERENT++

‘[…] because I can sign and I am the same as the other people there. And it is interesting that every day is different.’

Example 14

chapter 6 (p. 142): ONE DEAF SAY CURIOUS INDEX+f,hi

Taken from Laurence, 01:07

As the context for this example was already given above (cf. example 2, chapter 4), it is not provided here again.

Example 15

chapter 6 (p. 142): [...] WITH FRIEND FOUR DEAF PERSON

Taken from Laurence, 00:08

As the context for this example was already given above (cf. example 6a, chapter 4), it is not provided here again.

Example 16

chapter 6 (p. 142): index-me DEAF

Taken from Fergus D., 02:25

"engine" open_______________________ "off, off, off"____________________
ENGINE ENGINE-LOCATED-THERE HOW REMOVE-PARTS-OF-ENGINE++ OFF

"hard"______ closed, forward_______ "I"____ "help" "deaf"
HARD-WORK SMALL-NARROW-OBJECT index-me HELP FIX UP index-me DEAF

closed, tense, bilabial__________________ open, teeth clenched "long" "all"
FIX-UP REMOVE-PARTS-OF-ENGINE++++ SHAPE-OF-ENGINE LONG ALL

open_________________ "not" "finished"
index-me LOOK-AT-lo-fr NOT FINISH

'I looked at where the engine was located and removed several parts of the engine. [It was] hard work [because of] the small narrow objects. I am deaf and I helped [my mechanic friend] fixing up [the car] and removing parts of the engine. That took a long time but when I looked [at the car] it was still not finished.'

Notes

1. The terms "signed language" and "sign language" are used interchangeably in the remainder of this book as they are synonymous.
2. LBG = Lautsprachbegleitende Gebärden. While DGS manual signs are used, the rules of spoken German grammar are applied.
3. RTÉ is the first television channel in Ireland comparable to the BBC channel group in the UK.
4. Further information on deaf communities is provided in chapter 5.3.
5. An example from Bambara is the lexeme 'thank you'. A man, irrespective of the interlocutor's sex, has to use the lexeme *nbá*, while a woman, also irrespective of the interlocutor's sex, has to use *nsé*. This is not to be confused with grammatical gender.
6. There are different reasons for signs across sign languages to be related. Firstly, the two sign languages themselves may be related historically, as ASL and LSF, for example. However, signs from different unrelated sign languages often show striking similarities as well. These are due to a shared iconicity that is especially well expressed in the visual-gestural modality (cf. chapter 2.4). Moreover, language contact with the majority spoken language in a country might cause sign languages surrounded by the same spoken language to become increasingly similar (Johnston & Schembri 2007). Finally, the growing impact of ASL internationally is sometimes mentioned as a reason for a lexical overlap between different sign languages. They might simply have borrowed signs from ASL.
7. The ASL sign RESTAURANT, e.g., is formed with the R-handshape from the American manual alphabet.
8. If not indicated differently, the information in this section is taken from Matthews' book, esp. from pp. 58–114.
9. Figures 2.26 and 2.27 are reprinted with kind permission from the author.
10. The Milan Congress was an international conference of educators of the deaf at which the introduction of the oral method to deaf schools around the world was decided. The only opposing members, thus favouring sign language as medium of instruction in deaf schools, were from the United States and Britain.
11. All pictures from Ó Baoill and Matthews (2000) are reprinted with kind permission from the authors.
12. For a detailed description of the sociolinguistic setting and linguistic set-up of village sign languages, the reader is referred to, e.g., Johnson (1991), Nonaka (2004), Zeshan (2007), Nyst (2007; 2012), Schwager & Zeshan (2008).
13. The parameters determining signs in sign phonology are location, handshape and movement. More recent accounts of sign phonology add two more

parameters, namely orientation and non-manuals. This issue is elaborated on in section 2.5. For a detailed account of sign phonology the reader is referred to, e.g., Stokoe (1960), Sandler (2003), Sandler & Lillo-Martin (2006) and Brentari (2012).

14. It should be mentioned though that this claim refers to morphology only. Keller acknowledges a tripartite distinction of sign language verbs on functional semantic grounds.
15. For a detailed description of classifier constructions in sign languages the reader is referred to Emmorey (ed.) (2003). The topic will also be commented on briefly in the following.
16. It should be emphasized however, that sign phonology is not exclusively simultaneous. References to the sequentiality of sign phonology can be found e.g. in Liddell & Johnson (1989). Sandler (1989) proposes a rather balanced phonological model with respect to simultaneity and sequentiality.
17. The role of non-manual features in phonology is briefly touched upon in chapter 2.6 as well.
18. This has usually been called "aspect" in sign linguistics. However, I argue that these inflections are actually aktionsart inflections. The matter is discussed in further detail in chapter 6.
19. For a detailed analysis cf. chapter 3.
20. In this case, "subject" is used as a neutral term not referring to the syntactic function of subject.
21. Again, the term "predicate" does not refer to the syntactic function of predicates but is used neutrally.
22. The usual abbreviation for Israeli Sign Language is *ISL*. However, the in this book often used abbreviation for Irish Sign Language is also *ISL*. Thus, in order not to confuse the reader, I have chosen to use the abbreviation *IsSL* for Israeli Sign Language. The reader should be aware that this abbreviation is not used in other publications.
23. The figure first appeared in Sutton-Spence & Woll. 1999 [2006]. *The Linguistics of British Sign Language*. Cambridge: Cambridge University Press. The images are reprinted with kind permission from the authors and Cambridge University Press.
24. The expression "toward the subject" refers to the location of the subject in the signing space. The dynamics of verb agreement realized in spatial syntax were outlined in chapter 2.1.
25. The topic of pronouns in sign languages is also further elaborated on in chapter 6.1.4.
26. The figure first appeared in Pfau & Quer. 2010. Nonmanuals: their grammatical and prosodic roles. In Brentari (ed.) *Sign Languages*. Cambridge: Cambridge

University Press. The images are reprinted with kind permission from the authors and Cambridge University Press.

27. The transcription ")(" for indicating the sucking in of cheeks was used in the original.
28. Copyright © 1980 by Mouton de Gruyter. Reprinted with permission.
29. 'le' was used by the authors to indicate lowered eyebrows.
30. "whq" stands for the non-manual marker for WH-questions here.
31. The figure first appeared in Sandler & Lillo-Martin. 2006. *Sign Language and Linguistic Universals*. Cambridge: Cambridge University Press. The images are reprinted with kind permission from the authors and Cambridge University Press.
32. Additionally, Pfau and Quer (2007) claim that DGS relative clauses may be accompanied by a body lean towards the locus of the antecedent of the relative.
33. 're' was chosen to mean 'raised eyebrows'.
34. They observed that if an antecedent is mentioned in the preceding linguistic context, it is not marked by a squint later on.
35. In sign languages, another form of cliticization, namely coalescence, exists, too. The reader is referred to Sandler & Lillo-Martin (2006:248 f.) for further information.
36. For further information on the other four cases, cf. Hohenberger & Happ (2001:167 ff.).
37. Although the following discussion is exclusively concerned with mouth actions, spreading has been observed for other non-manuals such as negative headshakes or question markers.
38. This theory is based on a Prosodic Phonology model as used, e.g., by Sandler (1999) and Nespor and Sandler (1999).
39. For further information on this topic cf. Leeson and Grehan (2004:44 ff).
40. All information on the SOI is taken from Leeson (2008).
41. Children at St. Mary's and St. Joseph's usually start primary school at the age of four and finish at the age of 14. Post-primary education spans a period of approximately four years.
42. The second step was calculating the correlation between word classes and mouth actions.
43. No interlinear morpheme translation is provided for these examples because of the gestural component that could not easily be represented.
44. This relation of semantic congruence has been described by other researchers, such as Baker and Van den Bogaerde (2008) or Emmorey et al. (2005), e.g., for bilingual communication situations.

45. Formal criteria do not necessarily refer to complete formal identity of sign and spoken language items but rather to categorical similarities and differences concerning word classes or morphologically overlapping forms, for instance.
46. "Manual" here refers to the conventional gloss associated with a manual, which in turn is often determined by the associated mouthing. Moreover, transcription conventions often play an important role for the relation between a manual sign and its gloss. However, I have chosen to use "manual" instead of "gloss" in the following description of mouthing types.
47. In direct opposition to TYPE 3a are English prepositional verbs that are only accompanied by the mouthed preposition as LIFT-OFF and "off". These examples are much rarer than TYPE 3a and considered an exception from the general rule that the most salient part of a construction is mouthed.
48. For more information cf. chapter 5.3 and Mohr (2012).
49. In fact, even some of the cited examples were not transcribed like this in the ELAN files. I cited them from my own notes.
50. Acknowledgement: From "The visual-gestural modality and beyond". In *Sign Language and Linguistics* 15 (2012) pp. 185–211. With kind permission by John Benjamins Publishing Company, Amsterdam/Philadelphia. www.benjamins.com
51. It should be kept in mind however, that mostly lexical signs were considered for the sociolinguistic as well as for the linguistic analysis. Hence, the figures might be slightly biased with respect to this point. A few cases of spread prepositions to adjacent verbs or numerals to adjacent nouns hint at the fact that in few cases, function words might spread to content words. These findings are in line with findings for other sign languages that have been investigated regarding this issue.
52. Acknowledgement: From "The visual-gestural modality and beyond". In *Sign Language and Linguistics* 15 (2012) pp. 185–211. With kind permission by John Benjamins Publishing Company, Amsterdam/Philadelphia. www.benjamins.com
53. Brown Thomas is an Irish retail store which is now part of the Wittington Investment Group including Selfridges in the UK and Holt Renfrew in Canada.
54. The picture only shows the beginning of the fingerspelling, or rather the transition from c. to h. This is simply to give an impression of what the fingerspelling looks like as the whole word could not be shown in pictures.
55. Crasborn et al. (2008) mention four different types of mouth gestures in their study. Reasons for differentiating only three distinct types are given at the end of this section.
56. This also relates to the overall storyline as the signer described the trouble he had with his car and the engine not working.

57. This is the fourth type of mouth gesture as mentioned by Crasborn et al. (2008) which was excluded from the mouth gesture typology introduced here.
58. I want to thank my reviewer who indicated an error in transcription of the sign to me.
59. Another issue that should be mentioned in this context is the exaggerated size of the mouthings used in order to impersonate the hearing child's mouth movements. This, however, is probably a story-telling technique that is not relevant for the current investigation.
60. Thank you for my reviewer for this comment.
61. These figures exclude more marginal cases in which the spreading was not clearly visible.
62. This should be kept in mind when looking at figure 5.8.
63. For further reading on this matter cf. for example Emmorey et al. (2005), Baker & Van den Bogaerde (2008).
64. In this category, three signers (Michelle, Sarah Jane and Sean) were counted double as they had given two different modes of communication at home. These can be seen in Table 1.
65. The other cornerstone is deaf residential schools (Woll & Ladd 2003).
66. Woll & Ladd (2003:152, f.) establish four different kinds of Deaf communities in their paper: "suppressing communities" in which Deaf community life is organized separately from hearing community life, "assimilating communities" which arise in most non-industrialized communities with a high incidence of deafness, "single communities" in which the socioeconomic status and educational achievements of Deaf people are largely equivalent to those of hearing people and where hearing people have a considerable knowledge of sign language, and "integrated communities" in which the Deaf community is integrated to a greater or lesser extent within the hearing community.
67. Endocentric compounds usually consist of a head that determines the basic meaning of the construction. Most English compounds are right-headed such as *greenhouse* in which *house* functions as the head and *green* as the modifier of this head. Moreover, the head also determines the word class of the compound. Exocentric compounds however, do not possess a (expressed) head and their meaning is totally unrelated to its constituent parts, as in *skinhead*, for example.
68. Terminology is rather vague in this respect and varies between different approaches put forth by different researchers. In line with Sasse (1993b) and Haspelmath (2001) I consider the terms "word class" and "part-of-speech" to be synonymous.
69. Other categories closely related to personal pronouns are number and strong-weak distinctions. For further reference, the reader is referred to Sasse (1993b) and Helmbrecht (2004).

70. The cognitive classification of the extra-linguistic world varies in different cultures and hence causes a different categorization of words in different languages.

71. Semantically, there are a number of entity types that while treated as nouns in the familiar Indo-European languages, are realized as verbs or deverbal nominalizations in the languages of Australia and North America. Evans (2000:711) cites mostly kin terms, body parts and other part terms and ephemeral entities as examples of this phenomenon. Especially with respect to lexemes denoting ephemeral or dynamic features of the landscape, there are various languages in which many of these words are expressed as verbs. Thus, lexemes like *billabong*, *thunder*, *lightning* and so on are perceived to be of processual rather than stative nature in these languages and are consequently realized as verbs (one example is *kaboyo*= 'it-water-lies' = 'billabong' in Mayali (an Australian language from the Gunwingguan language family)).

72. The seven types are: **MOTION** e.g. verbs of motion like *go*, **AFFECT** e.g. verbs like *hit*, **GIVING** e.g. verbs like *donate*, **CORPOREAL** e.g. verbs like *laugh*, **OBJECTS** e.g. nouns like *tree*, **KIN** e.g. kinship terms like *son*, **DIMENSION** e.g. items like *deep*, **COLOUR** e.g. colour terms like *white*, **VALUE** e.g. items like *good*. For more detailed information, the reader is referred to Dixon (1982:12 ff.).

73. Taylor (1989) subsumes word classes, parts-of-speech and syntactic categories under the label "grammatical categories". For problematic issues with respect to the use of terminology cf. Rauh (2010).

74. This view however is doubted by several linguists, one of which is Croft (2000) who considers this to be an exaggerated claim.

75. Morphological markers providing information on the relation between two nouns in an NP may also occur as in Russian (possessor of another noun) or Hebrew (being possessed by another noun) (Evans 2000) also exist, but cannot be commented on here for spatial restrictions.

76. The fact that all linguistic levels have to be considered for a clear word class distinction is of course also supported by other researchers, such as Knobloch & Schaeder (2000), for example.

77. It can however be stated that the degree of compound friendliness varies between individual sign languages. Thus, Zeshan (2002) mentions ASL to be relatively compound friendly, while IPSL, e.g., is not. For further information the reader is also referred to Meir (2012).

78. Person distinctions in sign languages are discussed in more detail in the paragraph below on pronominal systems.

79. As is apparent from this statement, Erlenkamp suggests that syntactic categories and lexical classes are not equal in DGS. In her analysis, the members of the syntactic category of multifunctional signs can be divided into different lexical classes.

80. It should be mentioned that the term “pointer” is a generic term in this context as it refers to both pointers and zone indeces. The first indicate singular number while the latter mark the plural.
81. For a more detailed discussion of the issue of iconicity in sign languages cf. chapter 2.
82. As these parameters are very general, it is obvious that not all of them are applicable to the same extent to all languages. Isolating languages like Chinese, e.g. can only resort to distribution as formal parameter since they lack category identifying morphology (cf. chapter 6.1.3).
83. There is no interlinear morpheme translation in these examples as the language change within the sentences could not be adequately expressed.
84. While it has often been stated that sign language verbs inflect for aspect, I think the appropriate term here is aktionsart as the category expressed rather refers to the manner in which an action is carried out, rather than to its temporal structure.
85. At this point it should also be mentioned that a zero-subject as in (10) usually entails a 1sg/1pl subject (Leeson, p.c.) in ISL.
86. The idea of interpreting transfer as movement has also been tackled in section 6.2.1 already.
87. For a detailed account of backwards verbs cf. Müller de Quadros & Quer (2008).
88. The multifunctionality of aktionsart verbs 2 is not denied. However, the degree of syntactic indeterminacy seems to be greater in multifunctional signs.
89. In that respect, their findings are opposed to Fowler and Heaton’s (2006) results indicating that there are onomatopoeia in BSL.
90. This would be an alternative explanation for the high frequency of mouth gestures with verbs.
91. However, this analysis does not assume as high a degree of multifunctionality as Erlenkamp (2000), as there are four more lexical categories besides multinfunctional signs.
92. The syntactic categories then correlate with the lexical classes of ISL as shown in figure 6.2.
93. For further reference the reader is referred to Dik (1997:61).
94. Bank et al. (2011:265) make this claim with reference to frequent signs.
95. The class of ideophones is extremely structurally marked so that it is singled out by this criterion. Moreover, correlations with mouth actions could not be calculated here as it is constituted by mouth gestures only.
96. For the interested reader, fingerspellings were included in the following list.
97. Words in single quotes indicate a gesture.

98. This is the last sign of the narrative, thus the 10 seconds preceding the sign are provided here.
99. This is example 7b.
100. For continuation cf. example 5a.

References

Aarons, Debra. 1994. *Aspects of the syntax of American Sign Language*. PhD dissertation, Boston University.

Aboh, Enoch O./Pfau, Roland/Zeshan, Ulrike. 2005. When a Wh-Word is Not aWh-Word: The Case of Indian Sign Language. In: Bhattacharya, T. (ed.) *The Yearbook of South Asian Languages and Linguistics*. Berlin: Mouton de Gruyter, 11–43.

Adam, Meike/Iversen,Wiebke/Wilkinson, Erin/Morford, Jill P. 2007. Meaning on the one and on the other hand. Iconicity in native vs. foreign sign languages. In: Tabakowska, Elizabieta/Ljungberg, Christina/Fischer, Olga (eds.) *Insistent Images*. Amsterdam: John Benjamins, 209–225.

Adone, Dany/Bauer, Anastasia/Mohr, Susanne. 2009. Mouthing and mouth gestures in a young sign language. Paper presented at the Nonmanuals in Sign Languages Workshop, Frankfurt a. M.

Aikhenvald, Alexandra. 2006. Serial verb constructions in a typological perspective. In: Aikhenvald, Alexandra/Dixon, Robert M. W. (eds.) *Serial verb constructions: A cross-linguistic typology*. Oxford: Oxford University Press, 1–87.

Anward, Jan. 2000. A dynamic model of part-of-speech differentiation. In: Comrie, Bernard/Vogel, Petra M. (eds.) *Approaches to the typology of word classes*. Berlin: Mouton de Gruyter, 3–45.

Aronoff, Mark/Meir, Irit/Padden, Carol/Sandler, Wendy. 2003. Classifier Constructions and Morphology in Two Sign Languages. In: Emmorey, Karen (ed.) *Perspectives on Classifier Constructions in Sign Languages*. London: Psychology Press, 53–84.

Aronoff, Mark/Meir, Irit/Padden, Carol/Sandler, Wendy. 2005. Morphological universals and the sign language type. In: Booij, Geert/Marle, Jan van (eds.) *Yearbook of Morhology 2004*. Amsterdam: Kluwer Academic Publishers, 19–39.

Baker, Mark C. 1988. *Incorporation*. Chicago and London: The University of Chicago Press.

Baker, Mark C. 2003. *Lexical Categories: Verbs, Nouns and Adjectives*. Cambridge: Cambridge University Press.

Baker, Anne/Bogaerde, Beppie van den. 2008. Code-mixing in signs and words in input to and output from children. In: Plaza-Pust, Carolina/Morales-López, Esperanza (eds.) *Sign Bilingualism: language development, interaction, and maintenance in sign language contact situations*. Amsterdam/Philadelphia: John Benjamins, 1–28.

Bank, Richard/Crasborn, Onno/Hout, Rouland van. 2011. Variation in mouth actions with manual signs in Sign Language of the Netherlands (NGT). In: *Sign Language & Linguistics* 14(2), 248–270.

Battison, Robbin. 1978. *Lexical Borrowing in American Sign Language.* MD: Linstock.

Bellugi, Ursula/Klima, Edward S./Siple, Patricia. 1975. Remembering in signs. In: *Cognition* 3, 93–125.

Benedicto, Elena/Brentari, Diane. 2004. Where Did All The Arguments Go? Argument Changing Properties of Classifiers in ASL. In: *Natural Language and Linguistic Theory* 22, 743–810.

Benveniste, Emile. 1966. *Problèmes de linguistique générale.* Paris: Gallimard.

Bickmore, Lee. 1996. Bantu tone spreading and displacement as alignment and minimal misalignment. In: *Rutgers Optimality Archive* (http://roa.rutgers.edu), Philadelphia.

Blench, Roger (ed.). 2004. *Bura grammar for a beginner.* Bura Language and Bible Translation Project 2004.

Blench, Roger. 2009. The sensory world: ideophones in Africa and elsewhere. Draft circulated for comment.

Bolinger, Dwight. 1986. *Intonation and its Parts.* Palo Alto, CA: Stanford University Press.

Borer, Hagit. 2005a. *Structuring Sense: In Name Only.* Oxford: Oxford University Press.

2005b. *Structuring Sense: The Normal Course of Events.* Oxford: Oxford University Press.

Bouchard, Denis/Dubuisson, Colette/Parisot, Anne-Marie. 2005. Categorisation in Quebec Sign Language: Reflections on categorisation across modalities. In: Cohen, Henri/Lefèbvre, Claire (eds.) *Handbook of Categorization and Cognitive Science.* Amsterdam: Elsevier, 381–399.

Boyes-Braem, Penny. 2001. Functions of the mouthings in the signing of Deaf early and late learners of Swiss German Sign Language (DSGS). In: Boyes-Braem, Penny/Sutton-Spence, Rachel (eds.) *The Hands are the Head of the Mouth. The Mouth as Articulator in Sign Languages.* Hamburg: Signum, 99–131.

Boyes-Braem, Penny/Sutton-Spence, Rachel (eds.). 2001. *The Hands are the Head of the Mouth. The Mouth as Articulator in Sign Languages.* Hamburg: Signum.

Brennan, Mary. 1983. Marking Time in British Sign Language. In: Kyle, James G./ Woll, Bencie (eds.) *Language in Sign. An International Perspective on Sign Language.* London: Croom Helm, 10–31.

Brentari, Diane. 1998. *A Prosodic Model of Sign Language Phonology.* Cambridge, MA: MIT Press.

Brentari, Diane. 2007. Sign Language Phonology: Issues of Iconicity and Universality. In: Pizzuto, Elena/Pietrandrea, Paola/Simone, Raffaele (eds.) *Verbal and Signed Languages, Comparing Structures, Constructs and Methodologies.* Berlin: Mouton de Gruyter, 59–80.

Brentari, Diane. 2012. Phonology. In: Pfau, Roland/Steinbach, Markus/Woll, Bencie (eds.) *Sign Language. An International Handbook.* Berlin/New York: De Gruyter Mouton, 21–54.

Brenzinger, Matthias (ed.). 2007. *Language Diversity Endangered.* Berlin: Mouton de Gruyter.

Bußmann, Hadumod (ed.). 2002. *Lexikon der Sprachwissenschaft.* Stuttgart: Kroner.

Bynon, Theodora. 2004. Morphological typology and universals. In: Booij, Geert/ Lehmann, Christian/Mugdan, Joachim (eds.) *Morphology. An International Handbook on Inflection and Word-Formation.* Berlin/New York: Mouton de Gruyter, 1221–1231.

Chafe, Wallace L. 1982. Integration and involvement in speaking, writing and oral literature. In: Tannen, Deborah (ed.) *Spoken and written language: Exploring orality and literacy.* Norwood, NJ: Ablex, 35–53.

Cormier, Kearsy/Wechsler, Stephen/Meier Richard P. 1999. Locus Agreement in AmericanSign Language. In: Webelhut, Gert/Koenig, Jean-Pierre/Kathol, Andreas (eds.) *Lexical and constructional aspects of linguistic explanation.* Stanford, CA: CSLI Press, 215–229.

Cormier, Kearsy/Schembri, Adam/Woll, Bencie. 2010. Diversity across sign languages and spoken languages: Implications for language universals. In: *Lingua* 120(12), 2664–2667.

Cormier, Kearsy. 2007. Do all pronouns point? Indexicality of first person plural pronouns in BSL and ASL. In: Perniss, Pamela M./Pfau, Roland/Steinbach, Markus (eds.) *Visible Variation. Comparative Studies on Sign Language Structure.* Berlin/New York: Mouton de Gruyter, 63–101.

Coulter, Geoffrey. 1978. Raised Brows and Wrinkled Noses: The Grammatical Function of Facial Expression in Relative Clauses and Related Constructions. In: Caccamise, Frank/Hicks, Doin (eds.) *American Sign Language in a Bilingual, Bicultural Context. Proceedings of the Second National Symposium on Sign Language Research and Teaching.* Silver Spring: NAD, 65–74.

Crasborn, Onno/Kooij, Els van der. 1997. Relative Orientation in Sign Language Phonology. In: Coerts, Jane/Hoop, Helen de (eds.) *Linguistics in the Netherlands 1997.* Amsterdam: Benjamins, 37–48.

Crasborn, Onno/Kooij, Els van der/Waters, Dafydd/Woll, Bencie/Mesch, Johanna. 2008. Frequency distribution and spreading behaviour of different types of mouth actions in three sign languages. In: *Sign Language & Linguistics* 11(1),45–67.

Croft, William. 1984. Semantic and pragmatic correlates to syntactic categories. In: Testen, David/Mishra, Veena/Drogo, Joseph(eds.) *Papers from the Parasessionon Lexical Semantics*. Chicago: CLS, 53–70.

Croft, William. 1990. *Typology and Universals.* Cambridge: Cambridge University Press.

Croft, William. 1991. *Syntactic Categories and Grammatical Relations: The Cognitive Organisation of Information.* Chicago: Chicago University Press.

Croft, William. 2000. Parts of speech as language universals and as language particular categories. In: Vogel, Petra M./Comrie, Bernard (eds.) *Approaches to the Typology of Word Classes*. Berlin/New York: Mouton de Gruyter, 65–102.

Croft, William. 2007. Beyond Aristotle and gradience: A reply to Aarts. In: *Studies in Language* 31(2), 409–430.

Crystal, David. 1997 [1987]. *The Cambridge Encyclopedia of Language*. Cambridge: Cambridge University Press.

Dachkovsky, Svetlana/Sandler, Wendy. 2007. *Visual Intonation in the Prosody of a Sign Language*. Unpublished manuscript, University of Haifa.

Dimmendaal, Gerrit J. 2000. Number Marking and Noun Categorization in Nilo-Saharan Languages. In: *Anthropological Linguistics* 42(2), 214–261.

Dingemanse, Mark. 2011. *The Meaning and Use of Ideophones in Siwu.* PhD dissertation, Radboud University Nijmegen.

Dixon, Robert M.W. 1982. *Where have all the adjectives gone?* Berlin/New York: Mouton de Gruyter.

Drossard, Werner. 2009. Selbstbehauptung: das Überleben sprachlicher Minoritäten. *IABLIS*, 8 (online version).

Ebbinghaus, Horst/Heßmann, Jens. 1994. German Words in German Sign Language: Do They Tell Us Something about Sign Languages? In: Erting, Carol J./Johnson, Robert C./Smith, Dorothy L./Snider, Bruce D. (eds.) *The Deaf Way*. Washington, D.C.: Gallaudet University Press, 399–409.

Ebbinghaus, Horst/Heßmann, Jens. 2001. Sign Language as Multidimensional Communication: Why Manual Signs, Mouthings and Mouth Gestures are Three Different Things. In: Boyes-Braem, Penny/Sutton-Spence, Rachel (eds.) *The Hands are the Head of the Mouth. The Mouth as Articulator in Sign Languages*. Hamburg: Signum, 133–151.

Emmorey, Karen. 2002. *Language, cognition, and the brain: Insights from sign language research.* Mahwah, NJ: Lawrence Erlbaum Associates.

Ebbinghaus, Horst/Heßmann, Jens. 2002. *Language, cognition, and the brain: Insights from sign language research.* Mahwah, NJ: Lawrence Erlbaum Associates.

Emmorey, Karen (ed.). 2003. *Perspectives on classifier constructions in sign languages.* Mahwah, NJ: Lawrence Erlbaum Associates.

Engberg-Pedersen, Elisabeth. 1990. Pragmatics of Non-manual Behviour in Danish Sign Language. In: Edmondson, William/Karlsson, Fred (eds.) *SLR '87: Papers from the Fourth International Symposium on Sign Language Research.* Hamburg: Signum, 121–128.

Engberg-Pedersen, Elisabeth. 1993. *Space in Danish Sign Language.* Hamburg: Signum.

Erlenkamp, Sonja. 2000. *Syntaktische Kategorien und lexikalische Klassen: typologische Aspekte der Deutschen Gebärdensprache.* München: Lincom.

Evans, Nicholas. 2000. Word classes in the world's languages. In Booij, Geert/ Lehmann, Christian/Mugdan, Joachim (eds.) *Morphology. An International Handbook on Inflection and Word-Formation.* Berlin/New York: Mouton de Gruyter, 708–732.

Evans, Nicholas/Stephen C. Levinson. 2009. The myth of language universals: Language diversity and its importance for cognitive science. In: *Behavioural and brain sciences*, 32, 429–492.

Fischer, Renate/Leven, Regina. 2004. Deutsche Gebärdensprache. In: Booij, Geert/ Lehmann, Christian/Mugdan, Joachim (eds.) *Morphology. An International Handbook on Inflection and Word-Formation.* Berlin/New York: Mouton de Gruyter, 1554–1562.

Fischer, Renate/Kollien, Simon. 2009. Constructed Action und Mundgestik in DGS: Lautmalerei und synästhetische Symbolisierungsverfahren. In: *DAS ZEICHEN*, 464–478.

Flodlin, Mickey. 1994. *Signing Illustrated. The Complete Learning Guide.* New York: Berkley Publishing Group.

Fowler, David/Heaton, Mark. 2006. Onomatopoeia in British Sign Language? or The visuality/sensation of sound. In: Goodstein, Harvey (ed.) *The Deaf Way II Reader. Perspectives from the second international conference on Deaf culture.* Washington, D.C.: Gallaudet University Press, 241–244.

Frishberg, Nancy. 1976. *Some Aspects of the Historical Development of Signs in American Sign Language.* PhD dissertation, University of California, San Diego.

Gilley, Leoma. 2004. *Morphophonemic Orthographies in Fusional Languages. The Cases of Dinka and Shilluk.* Institute of African and Asian Studies, University of Khartoum and SIL International.

Glück, Susanne/Pfau, Roland. 1999. On classifying classification as a class of inflection in German Sign Language. In: Cambier-Langeveld, Tina/Liptak, Aniko/Redford, Michael (eds.) *Proceedings of ConSole 6.* Leiden: SOLE, 59–74.

Gomez-Imbert, Elsa/Kenstowicz, Michael. 2000. Barasana tone and accent. In: *International Journal of American Linguistics*, 66(4), 419–463.

Greenberg, Joseph H. 1963. Some universals of grammar with particular reference to the order of meaningful elements. In: Greenberg, Joseph H. (ed.) *Universals of Language*. Cambirdge, MA: MIT Press, 73–113.

Greenberg, Joseph H. 1986. Introduction. Some Reflections on *Pronominal Systems*. In: Wiesemann, Ursula (ed.) Pronominal systems. Tübingen: Gunter Narr, XVII–XXI.

Grinevald, Colette. 2000. A morphosyntactic typology of classifiers. In: Senft, Gunter(ed.) *Systems of nominal classification.* Cambridge: Cambridge University Press, 50–92.

Guerra-Curie, Anne-Marie P./Meier, Richard P./Walters, Keith. 2002. A crosslinguistic examination of the lexicons of four signed languages. In: Meier, Richard P./Cormier, Keary/Quinto-Pozos, David (eds.) *Modality and structure in signed and spoken languages*. Cambridge: Cambridge University Press, 224–235.

Gundel, Jeannette K. 1977. *The role of topic and comment in linguistic theory*. Bloomington, IN: Garland.

Harder, Rita. 1991. Incorporatie. In: Schermer, Trude/Fortgens, Connie/Harder, Rita/Nobel, Esther de (eds.) *De Neederlandse Gebarentaal.* Amsterdam: NSDSK/ Van Tricht, 119–124.

Haspelmath, Martin. 2001. Word Classes and Parts of Speech. In: Smelser, Neil J./ Baltes, Paul B.(eds.) *International Encyclopedia of the Social and Behavioural Sciences*. Amsterdam: Pergamon, 16538–45.

Haspelmath, Martin. 2010. Comparative concepts and descriptive categories in cross-linguistic studies. In: *Language*, 86, 663–687.

Hayward, Richard J. 2000. Afroasiatic. In: Heine, Bernd/Nurse, Derek (eds.) *African Languages. An Introduction.* Cambridge: Cambridge University Press, 74–98.

Heine, Bernd. 1997. *Possession: Cognitive Sources, Forces, Grammaticalisation.* Cambridge: Cambridge University Press.

Hellwig, Birgit. 2011. *A Grammar of Goemai.* Berlin: Mouton de Gruyter.

Hellwig, Birgit. 2010. Meaning and translation in linguistic fieldwork. In: *Studies in Language* 34(4), 802–831.

Hengeveld, Kees. 1992. Parts of speech. In: Fortescue, Michael D./Harder, Peter/ Kristofferson, Lars(eds.) *Layered structure and reference in a functional perspective. Papers from the Functional Grammar Conference in Copenhagen 1990.* Amsterdam: John Benjamins, 29–55.

Hengeveld, Kees/Rijkhoff, Jan/Siewierska, Anna. 2004. Parts-of-speech systems and word order. In: *Journal of Linguistics*, 40, 527–570.

Helmbrecht, Johannes. 2004. *Personal Pronouns – Form, Function and Grammaticalization.* Habilitationsschrift, Universität Erfurt.

Himmelmann, Nikolaus. 1987. *Morphosyntax und Morphologie - Die Ausrichtungsaffixe im Tagalog.* München: Fink.

Himmelmann, Nikolaus. 2008. Lexical categories and voice in Tagalog. In: Austin, Peter K./Musgrave, Simon (eds.) *Voice and Grammatical Relations in Austronesian Languages.* Stanford: CSLI, 247–293.

Hockett, Charles F. 1960. The origin of speech. *Scientific American*, 88–96.

Hohenberger, Annette/Happ, Daniela. 2001. The Linguistic Primacy of Signs over Mouthings: Evidence from Language Production in German Sign Language (DGS). In: Boyes-Braem, Penny/Sutton-Spence, Rachel (eds.) *The Hands are the Head of the Mouth. The Mouth as Articulator in Sign Languages.* Hamburg: Signum, 153–189.

Hopper, Paul J./Thompson, Sandra A. 1984. The discourse basis for lexical categories in universal grammar. In: *Language* 60, 703–752.

Hopper, Paul J./Thompson, Sandra A. 1985. The iconicity of the universal categories 'Noun' and 'Verb'. In: Haiman, John (ed.) *Iconicity in Syntax.* Amsterdam: John Benjamins, 151–183.

Howe, Neil/Strauss, William (eds.). 1992. *Generations: The History of America's Future. (1584 to 2069).* New York/London/Sydney/Tokyo: Harper Perennial.

Hulst, Harry van der. 1993. Units in the analysis of signs. In: *Phonology* 10, 209–242.

Hulst, Harry van der. 1995. The Composition of Handshapes. In: *University of Trondheim Working Papers in Linguistics* 23, 1–18.

Jackendoff, Ray. 1983. *Semantics and cognition.* Cambridge, MA: MIT Press.

Johnson, Robert E. 1991. Sign Language, Culture & Community in a Traditional Yucatec Maya Village. In: *Sign Language Studies* 73, 461–474.

Johnston, Trevor. 2001. Nouns and Verbs in Australian Sign Language: An Open and Shut Case? In: *Journal of Deaf Studies and Deaf Education* 6(4), 235–257.

Keller, Jörg. 1998. *Aspekte der Raumnutzung in der Deutschen Gebärdensprache.* Hamburg: Signum.

Keller, Jörg. 1999. Mundbilder in europäischen Gebärdensprachen. In: *DAS ZEICHEN* 13(37), 136–143.

Keller, Jörg. 2001. Multimodal Representations and the Linguistic Status of Mouthings in German Sign Language (DGS). In: Boyes-Braem, Penny/Sutton-Spence, Rachel (eds.) *The Hands are the Head of the Mouth. The Mouth as Articulator in Sign Languages*. Hamburg: Signum, 191–230.

Kinkade, M. Dale. 1983. Salish evidence against the universality of 'noun' and 'verb'. In:*Lingua* 60, 25–40.

Klima, Edward S./Bellugi, Ursular. 1979. *The Signs of Language*. Cambridge, MA: Harvard University Press.

Knobloch, Clemens/Schaeder, Burkhard. 2000. Kriterien für die Definition von Wortarten. In Booij, Geert/Lehmann, Christian/Mugdan, Joachim (eds.) *Morphology. An International Handbook on Inflection and Word-Formation.* Berlin/New York: Mouton de Gruyter, 674–692.

Kooij, Els van der. 2002. *Phonological Categories in Sign Language of the Netherlands: The Role of Phonetic Implementation and Iconicity.* Utrecht: LOT.

Kutscher, Silvia. 2007. Non-verbale Prädikation in der Deutschen Gebärdensprache: Probleme der Abgrenzung von Attribution und Prädikation in einer kopulalosen Sprache. In: Geist, Ljudmila/Rothstein, Björn (eds.) *Kopulaverben und Kopulasätze*. Tübingen: Max Niemeyer, 91–113.

Kutscher, Silvia. 2010. Ikonizität und Indexikalität im gebärdensprachlichen Lexikon – Zur Typologie sprachlicher Zeichen. In: *Zeitschrift für Sprachwissenschaft* 29(1), 79–110.

Kyle, James G./Woll, Bencie (eds.). 1985. *Sign Language: The Study of Deaf People and their language.* Cambridge: Cambridge University Press.

Langacker, Ronald W. 1991. *Foundations of Cognitive Grammar*. Stanford, CA: Stanford University Press.

Leeson, Lorraine. 2008. Quantum Leap. Leveraging the Signs of Ireland Digital Corpus in Irish Sign Language/English Interpreter Training. In: *The Sign Language Translator and Interpreter* 2(2), 149–176.

Leeson, Lorraine/Grehan, Carmel. 2004. To the Lexicon and Beyond: The Effect of Gender Variation on Irish Sign Language. In: Herreweghe, Mieke van and Vermeerbergen, Myriam (eds.) *To the Lexicon and Beyond: Sociolinguistics in European Deaf Communities*. Washington, D.C.: Gallaudet University Press, 39–73.

LeMaster, Barbara. 1990. *The Maintenance and loss of female and male signs in the Dublin deaf community.* PhD dissertation, University of California, Los Angeles.

LeMaster, Barbara/Dwyer, John P. 1991. Knowing and using female and male signs in Dublin. In: *Sign Language Studies*, 73, 361–396.

Lewin, Donna/Schembri, Adam. 2009. Adverbial mouth gestures in British Sign Language: A case study of tongue protrusion in BSL narratives. Paper presented at the NISL workshop, Frankfurt a. M.

Lewin, Donna/Schembri, Adam. 2011. Mouth gestures in British Sign Language: A case study of tongue protrusion in BSL narratives. In: *Sign Language & Linguistics* 14(1), 94–114.

Liddell, Scott. 1980. *American Sign Language Syntax.* The Hague: Mouton.

Liddel, Scott/Johnson, Robert. 1987. An analysis of spatial-locative predicates in American Sign Language. Paper presented at the fourth International Symposium on Sign Language Research, Lappeenrata, Finland.

Liddel, Scott/Johnson, Robert. 1989. American Sign Language: The phonological base. In: *Sign Language Studies* 64, 197–277.

Lillo-Martin, Diane. 2005. Syntactic Categories in Signed versus Spoken Languages. In: Cohen, Henri/Lefèbvre, Claire (eds.) *Handbook of Categorization and Cognitive Science*. Amsterdam: Elsevier, 401–421.

Matthews, Patrick A. 1996. *The Irish Deaf Community, Volume 1. Survey Report, history of education, language and culture*. Dublin: The Linguistics Institute of Ireland.

McGurk, Harry/MacDonald, John. 1976. Hearing lips and seeing voices. In: *Nature* 264, 746–748.

Meir, Irit. 2001. Verb classifiers as noun incorporation in Israeli Sign Language. In: Booij, Geert/Marle, Jan van (eds.) *Yearbook of Morphology 1999*. Dordrecht: Kluwer Academic Publishers, 299–319.

Meir, Irit. 2002. A Cross-modality Perspective on Verb Agreement. In: *Natural Language and Linguistic Theory* 20(2), 413–450.

Meir, Irit. 2004. Question and Negation in Israeli Sign Language. In: *Sign Language & Linguistics* 7(2), 97–124.

Meir, Irit. 2012. Word classes and word formation. In: Pfau, Roland/Steinbach, Markus/Woll, Bencie (eds.) *Sign Language. An International Handbook.* Berlin/New York: De Gruyter Mouton, 77–112.

Meir, Irit/Sandler, Wendy. 2008. *A Language in Space: The Story of Israeli Sign Language*. New York: Lawrence Erlbaum.

Meir, Irit/Aronoff, Mark/Sandler, Wendy/Padden, Carol. 2010. Sign Languages and *Compounding*. In: Scalise, Sergio/Vogel Irene (eds), Compounding. Benjamins, 301–322.

Moessner, Lilo. 2003. *Diachronic English Linguistics. An Introduction*. Tübingen: Narr.

Mohr, Susanne. 2007. *Sign Languages as Natural Languages – The Linguistic Design Features*. MA thesis, RWTH Aachen University.

Mohr, Susanne. 2012. The visual-gestural modality and beyond. Mouthings as a language contact phenomenon in Irish Sign Language. *Sign Language & Linguistics* 15(2), 185–211.

Nadolske, Marie A./Rosenstock, Rachel. 2007. Occurrence of mouthings in American Sign Language: A preliminary study. In: Perniss, Pamela M./Pfau, Roland/Steinbach, Markus (eds.) *Visible Variation. Comparative Studies on Sign Language Structure*. Berlin/New York: Mouton de Gruyter, 36–61.

Nanny, Max/Fischer, Olga (eds.). 1999. *Form Miming Meaning: Iconicity in Language and Literature*. Amsterdam: John Benjamins.

Neidle, Carol/Kegl, Judy/MacLaughlin, Dawn/Bahan, Benjamin/Lee, Robert G.(eds.). 2000. *The Syntax of American Sign Language: Functional Categories and Hierarchical Structure*. Cambridge, MA: MIT Press.

Nespor, Marina/Sandler, Wendy. 1999. *Prosody in Israeli Sign Language.* In: *Language & Speech* 42(2&3), 143–176

Newman, Paul(ed.). 2000. *The Hausa Language. An Encyclopaedic Reference Grammar*. New Haven, CT: Yale University Press.

Nobe, Shuichi. 1996. *Representational Gestures, Cognitive Rhythms, and Acoustic Aspects of Speech: A Network/Threshold Model of Gesture Production.* Unpublished PhD dissertation, University of Chicago.

Nonaka, Angela M. 2004. The forgotten endangered languages: Lessons on the importance of remembering from Thailand's Ban Khor Sign Language. In: *Language in Society* 33, 737–767.

Nyst, Victoria. 2007. *A Descriptive Analysis of Adamorobe Sign Language (Ghana)*. Utrecht: LOT.

Nyst, Victoria. 2012. Shared Sign Languages. In: Pfau, Roland/Steinbach, Markus/Woll, Bencie (eds.) *Sign Language. An International Handbook*. Berlin/New York: De Gruyter Mouton, 552–573.

O'Baoill, Donall P./Matthews, Patrick A.(eds.). 2000. *The Irish Deaf Community, Volume 2. The Structure of Irish Sign Language*. Dublin: The Linguistics Institute of Ireland.

Padden, Carol. 1980. The deaf community and the culture of deaf people. In: Baker, Charlotte/Battison, Robbin (eds.) *Sign language and deaf community. Essays in honor of William C. Stokoe*. Silver Spring: NAD, 89–104.

Padden, Carol. 1988. *Interaction of morphology and syntax in American Sign Language*. Garland: Garland.

Peirce, Charles S. 1931–1958. *Collected Papers (8 vols.).* Cambridge, MA: Harvard University Press.

Petronio, Karen/Lillo-Martin, Diane. 1997. Wh-Movement and the position of Spec CP: evidence from American Sign Language. In: *Language* 73, 18–57.

Pfau, Roland. 2005. Phrasal Layers and Prosodic Spreading in Sign Languages. Paper presented at the SIGNA VOLANT Workshop, Milan.

Pfau, Roland. 2009. On Spreading: Domains and Hierarchies. Paper presented at the NISL Workshop, Frankfurt a. M.

Pfau, Roland/Steinbach, Markus. 2005. Relative Clauses in German Sign Language: Extra position and Reconstruction, Vol. 2. In Bateman, Leah/Ussery, Cherlon (eds.) *Proceedings of the North East Linguistic Society (NELS35)*. Amherst, MA: GLSA, 507–521.

Pfau, Roland/Quer, Josep. 2010. Nonmanuals: their grammatical and prosodic roles. In: Brentari, Diane (ed.) *Sign Languages*. Cambridge: Cambridge University Press, 381–402.

Pietrandrea, Paola. 2002. Iconicity and arbitrariness in Italian Sign Language. In: *Sign Language Studies* 2(3), 296–321.

Pizzuto, Elena/Volterra, Virginia. 2000. Iconicity and Transparency in Sign Languages: A Cross-Linguistic Cross-Cutural View. In: Emmorey, Karen/ Lane, Harlan H. (eds.) *The Signs of Language Revisited: An Anthologyin Honor of Ursula Bellugi and Edward Klima*. Mahwah, NJ: Lawrence Erlbaum, 261–286.

Poizner, Howard/Bellugi, Ursula/Tweney, Ryan D. 1981. Processing of Formational, Semantic and Iconic Information in American Sign Language. In: *Journal of Experimental Psychology: Human Perception and Performance* 7, 1146–1159.

Poplack, Shana/Meechan, Marjory. 1998. How languages fit together in code mixing. *International Journal of Bilingualism* 2(2), 127–138.

Prillwitz, Siegmund. 1985. *Grammatik der Deutschen Gebärdensprache*. Hamburg: Forschungsstelle Deutsche Gebärdensprache.

de Quadros, Ronice M./Quer, Josep. 2008. Back to back(wards) and moving on: on agreement, auxiliaries and verb classes in sign languages. In: de Quadros, Ronice M.(eds.) *Sign Languages: spinning and unraveling the past, present and future. TISLR9, forty five papers and three posters from the 9th Theoretical Issues in Sign Language Research Conference, Florianopolis, Brazil, December 2006*. Petropolis/RJ: Editora Arara Azul, 530–551.

Rainò, Päivi. 2001. Mouthings and mouth gestures in Finnish Sign Language. In: Boyes-Braem, Penny/Sutton-Spence, Rachel (eds.) *The Hands are the Head of the Mouth. The Mouth as Articulator in Sign Languages*. Hamburg: Signum, 41–49.

Rauh, Gisa. 2010. *Syntactic Categories. Their Identification and Description in Linguistic Theories.* Oxford: Oxford University Press.

Reagan, Timothy G. 2010. *Language Policy and Planning for Sign Languages.* Washington, D.C.: Gallaudet University Press.

Reuse, Willem de. 1999. Noun Incorporation. In: Brown, Keith/Miller, Jim (eds.) *Concise Encyclopedia of Grammatical Categories*. Amsterdam: Elsevier, 252–258.

Rijkhoff, Jan. 2000. When can a language have adjectives? An implicational universal. In: Vogel, Petra M./Comrie, Bernard (eds.) *Approaches to the Typology of Word Classes*. Berlin/New York: Mouton de Gruyter, 217–257.

Rijkhoff, Jan. 2007. Word classes. In: *Language and Linguistic Compass* 1(6), 709–726.

Russo, Tommasso. 2005. A Cross-cultural, Cross-linguistic Analysis of Metaphors in Two Italian Sign Language Registers. In: *Sign Language Studies* 5, 333–359.

Sandler, Wendy. 1989. *Phonological Representation of the Sign: Linearity and Nonlinearity in American Sign Language.* Dordrecht: Foris Publications.

Sandler, Wendy. 1999. Cliticization and prosodic words in a sign language. In: Hall, T. Alan/Kleinhenz, Ursula (eds.) *Studies on the phonological word.* Amsterdam: John Benjamins, 223–254.

Sandler, Wendy. 2003. Sign Language Phonology. In: Frawley, William (eds.) *The Oxford International Encyclopedia of Lingusitics*. Oxford: Oxford University Press.

Sandler, Wendy. 2009. Symbiotic symbolization by hand and mouth in sign language. In: *Semiotica* 174(1-4), 241–275.

Sandler, Wendy. 2012. Visual Prosody. In: Pfau, Roland/Steinbach, Markus/Woll, Bencie (eds.) *Sign Language. An International Handbook.* Berlin/New York: De Gruyter Mouton, 55–76.

Sandler, Wendy/Lillo-Martin, Diane (eds.). 2006. *Sign Language and Linguistic Universals*. Cambridge: Cambridge University Press.

Sapir, Edward. 1921. *Language*. Teddington: The Echo Library.

Sasse, Hans-Jürgen. 1993a. Das Nomen – eine universale Kategorie?In: *Sprachtypologische Universalienforschung* 46(3), 187–221.

Sasse, Hans-Jürgen. 1993b. Syntactic Categories and Subcategories. In Jacobs, Joachim/Stechow, Arnim von/Sternefeld, Wolfgang/Vennemann, Theo (eds.) *Syntax. Ein internationales Handbuch zeitgenössischer Forschung (HSK 9)*. Berlin/New York: Mouton de Gruyter, 646–686.

de Saussure, Ferdinand. 1989 [1968]. *Cours de Linguistique Générale (Édition Critique par Rudolf Engler)*. Wiesbaden: Otto Harrassowitz.

Schachter, Paul. 1985. Parts-of-speech systems. In: Shopen, Timothy (ed.) *Language typology and syntactic description (Volume I: Clause Structure)*. Cambridge: Cambridge University Press, 3–61.

Schuit, Joke. 2007. *The typological classification of sign language morphology*. MA thesis, Universiteit van Amsterdam.

Schuit, Joke. 2009. Verb agreement in Inuit Sign Language. Paper presented at the NAP-dag, Amsterdam.

Schwager, Waldemar/Zeshan, Ulrike. 2008. Word classes in sign languages. *Sign Language & Linguistics* 32(3), 509–545.

Selkirk, Elisabeth O. (ed.). 1984. *Phonology and Syntax. The Relation between Sound and Structure*. Cambridge, MA: MIT University Press.

Stassen, Leon. 1997. *Intransitive predication*. Oxford: Oxford University Press.

Stokoe, William C. 1960. Sign Language Structure: An Outline of the Visual Communication Systems of the American Deaf. In: *Studies in Linguistics. Occasional Papers*.

Storch, Anne. 2005. *The Noun Morphology of Western Nilotic*. Köln: Köppe.

Strixner, Stefan/Wolf, Serona. 2006 [2004]. *Kleines Wörterbuch der Gebärdensprache*. Wiesbaden: Marix Verlag GmbH.

Supalla, Ted. 1982. *Structure and acquisition of verbs of motion and location in American Sign Language*. PhD dissertation, University of California, San Diego.

Supalla, Ted. 1986. The classifier system in American Sign Language. In: Craig, Collette Grinevald (ed.) *Noun classes and categorization*. Philadelphia: John Benjamins, 181–214.

Supalla, Ted. 1990. Serial Verbs of Motion in ASL. In: Fischer, Susan D./Siple, Patricia (eds.) *Theoretical Issues in Sign Language Research, Vol. 1: Linguistics*. Chicago: University of Chicago Press., 127–152.

Sutton-Spence, Rachel/Day, Linda. 2001. Mouthings and Mouth Gestures in British Sign Language. In: Boyes-Braem, Penny/Sutton-Spence, Rachel (eds.) *The Hands are the Head of the Mouth. The Mouth as Articulator in Sign Languages*. Hamburg: Signum, 69–85.

Sutton-Spence, Rachel/Woll, Bencie (eds.). 2006 [1999]. *The Linguistics of British Sign Language*. Cambridge: Cambridge University Press.

Sze, Felix. 2009. Nonmanual markings for topic constructions in Hong Kong Sign Language. Paper presented at the NISL meeting, Frankfurt a. M.

Talmy, Leonard. 1985. Lexicalization patterns: semantic structure in lexical forms. In: Shopen, Timothy (ed.) *Language typology and syntactic description (Volume III: Grammatical catergories and the lexicon)*. Cambridge: Cambridge University Press, 57–149.

Tannen, Deborah. 1985. Relative focus on involvement and written discourse. In: Olson, David R./Torrance, Nancy/Hilyard, Angela (eds.) *Literacy, Language and Learning: The Nature and Consequences of Reading and Writing*. Cambridge: Cambridge University Press, 124–147.

Taub, Sarah. 2001. *Language from the Body: Iconicity and Metaphor in American Sign Language*. Cambridge: Cambridge University Press.

Thompson, Robin/Emmorey, Karen/Kluender, Robert. 2006. The relationship between eye gaze and verb agreement in American Sign Language: An eye-tracking study. In: *Natural Language & Linguistic Theory*, 24, 571–604.

Tsunoda, Tasaku. 2006. *Language Endangerment and Language Revitalization*. Berlin: Mouton de Gruyter.

Voghel, A. 2005. Phonologically identical noun-verb pairs in Quebec Sign Language (LSQ): Form and context. *Toronto Working Papers in Linguistics* 25, 68–75.

Vogt-Svendsen, Marit. 2001. A Comparison of Mouth Gestures and Mouthings in Norwegian Sign Language (NSL). In Boyes-Braem, Penny/Sutton-Spence, Rachel (eds.) *The Hands are the Head of the Mouth. The Mouth as Articulator in Sign Languages*. Hamburg: Signum, 9–40.

Westermann, Diedrich. 1907. *Grammatik der Ewe-Sprache*. Berlin: Dietrich Reimer.

Whaley, Lindsay J. (ed.). 1997. *Introduction to Typology. The Unity and Diversity of Language*. Thousand Oaks: Sage Publications.

Wierzbicka, Anna. 1996. *Semantics: Primes and Universals*. Oxford: Oxford University Press.

Wierzbicka, Anna. 2000. Lexical prototypes as a universal basis for crosslinguistic identification of "parts of speech". In: Vogel, Petra M./Comrie, Bernard (eds.) *Approaches to the Typology of Word Classes*. Berlin/New York: Mouton de Gruyter, 285–317.

Wilbur, Ronnie B. 1991. Intonation and focus in American Sign Language. Paper presented at ESCOL '90: the Seventh Eastern States Conference on Linguistics.

Wilbur, Ronnie B. 2010. The Event Visibility Hypothesis. In Brentari, Diane (ed.) *Sign Languages. A Cambridge Language Survey.* Cambridge, MA: Cambridge University Press, 355–380.

Wilcox, Sherman/Wilcox, Phyllis P. 1995. The Gestural Expression of Modality in ASL. In: Bybee, Joan L./Fleischman, S.(eds.) *Modality in Discourse and Grammar*. Amsterdam: John Benjamins, 135–162.

Wilcox, Sherman. 2004. Cognitive iconicity: Conceptual spaces, meaning and gesture in signed language research. In: Janzen, Terry (ed.) *Cognitive Linguistics: Special Issue: Cognitive approaches to signed language research.* Berlin: Mouton de Gruyter, 119–147.

Wilkinson, Erin L. 2009. *Typology of signed languages: differentiation through kinship terminology*. PhD dissertation, University of New Mexico.

Woll, Bencie. 1981. Question Structure in British Sign Language. In: Woll, Bencie/Kyle, James G./Deuchar, Margaret (eds.) *Perspectives on British Sign Language and Deafness.* London: Croom Helm, 136–149.

Woll, Bencie. 2001. The Sign that Dares to Speak its Name: Echo Phonology in British Sign Language (BSL). In: Boyes-Braem, Penny/Sutton-Spence, Rachel (eds.) *The Hands are the Head of the Mouth. The Mouth as Articulator in Sign Languages*. Hamburg: Signum, 87–98.

Woodward, James C. 1978. Historical bases of American Sign Language. In: Siple, Patricia (ed.) *Understanding language through sign language research.* New York: Academic Press, 333–348.

Yip, Moira. 2002. *Tone*. Cambridge: Cambridge University Press.

Zeshan, Ulrike. 2000. *Sign Language in Indo-Pakistan: A Description of a Signed Language*. Amsterdam: Benjamins.

Zeshan, Ulrike. 2002. Towards a notion of 'word' in sign languages. In: Dixon, Robert M. W./Aikhenvald, Alexandra (eds.) *Word. A cross-linguistic typology.* Cambridge: Cambridge University Press, 153–179.

Zeshan, Ulrike. 2004. Interrogative Constructions in Signed Languages: Cross-Linguistic Perspectives. In: *Language* 80, 7–39.

Zeshan, Ulrike. 2006. Negative and Interrogative Constructions in Sign Languages: A Case Study in Sign Language Typology. In: Zeshan, Ulrike (ed.) *Interrogative and Negative Constructions in Sign Languages*. Nijmegen: Ishara Press, 28–68.

Zeshan, Ulrike. 2008. Roots, leaves and branches – The typology of sign languages. In: de Quadros, Ronice M. (ed.) *Sign Languages: spinning and unraveling the past, present and future. TISLR9, forty five papers and three posters from the 9th Theoretical Issues in Sign Language Research Conference, Florianopolis, Brazil, December 2006*. Petropolis/RJ: Editora Arara Azul, 671–695.

Zwitserlood, Inge. 2003. Word formation below and above little x: Evidence from Sign Language of the Netherlands. In: Dahl, Anne/Bentzen, Kristine/Svenonius, Peter (eds.) *Nordlyd: Proceedings of the 19th Scandinavian Conference of Linguistics*. University of Tromsø: Septentrio Academic Publishing, 488–502.

Zwitserlood, Inge/Gijn, Ingeborg van. 2006. Agreement Phenomena in Sign Language of the Netherlands. In: Ackema, Peter/Brandt, Patrick/Schoorlemmer, Maaike/Weermann, Fred (eds.) *Arguments and Agreement*. Oxford: Oxford University Press, 195–229.

Index

adjective 52, 64, 86, 119, 121, 124, 149, 158

adverbial mouth gesture 52, 86–87

age 2, 66, 68–69, 93–95, 98, 102–112, 127, 142, 157, 162–163

age group 68–69, 102–111, 163

agreement 12–14, 18, 20, 22, 33, 48, 124–125, 129, 137, 139–140

aktionsart ditributive 137–138, 140–141, 143, 156

aktionsart intensive 128, 137–138, 140–141, 143, 156

aktionsart iterative 75, 129, 137–138, 140–141, 143, 156

aktionsart verb 12–20, 23, 33, 42, 53, 64, 73–75, 78, 80, 84, 92, 117–119, 121, 124–125, 128–129, 134, 139–140, 142, 145, 147–148, 151–156, 160–161, 164

American Sign Language (ASL) 2, 4, 13, 15, 19, 21–23, 33, 37–40, 42–43, 45, 49–52, 59–60, 75, 114, 127–130, 132, 155

aspect 23, 53, 75–76, 123–125, 128–129, 133, 141, 143

attributive 134, 142, 158

Australian Sign Language (Auslan) 40, 128–129

bare predicate 137, 144, 146, 156

bilingualism 6–8, 56, 112, 163

British Sign Language (BSL) 4, 32, 35, 48–50, 52–55, 59–60, 62–63, 92, 130, 135, 149

citation form 14, 17, 54, 160

classifier 14, 20–21, 73–74, 84, 92, 121, 134, 137, 142, 149, 160

code-switching 55, 62, 75–76, 110, 165

content word 80, 101, 104

conventional 15, 69, 84–86, 88, 92, 96, 149–151, 154

cross-linguistic 2, 21, 28, 38–39, 42–43, 49, 61, 89, 116–117, 119–120, 123–124, 126, 128–129, 132–133, 138

cross-modal 51, 109–110

deaf 4–12, 18, 51, 56–57, 66–67, 70, 76, 83, 94, 108, 111–112, 142–143, 163, 165

Deutschschweizer Gebärdensprache (DSGS) 59, 72, 80

disambiguation 51, 58–59, 96, 114, 146

distributional analysis 122

echo phonology 19, 51–55, 89, 91, 150

eye gaze 32–34, 58, 67, 131

facial expression 25, 28, 32, 34–39, 44–48, 53

fingerspelling 82, 92

focus 2, 4–5, 7, 22, 32, 42, 53, 55, 160–161

functional grammar 158, 161, 164

function word 79–80, 104

gender 2, 7–8, 10, 30, 93–95, 101–102, 104, 106–108, 112, 123–124, 129, 162–163
German Sign Language (DGS) 2, 6, 13, 19, 36, 42–45, 51–52, 56, 58–60, 128–130, 133, 142, 149, 154, 158
gesture 51–54, 69–70, 80, 85–91, 95, 99, 146, 149, 152–154
gloss 69, 71–72, 152
gradience 117–118, 120–123, 128
grammatical category 124

headshake 26, 28–29, 49
hearing 6–7, 11–12, 56–57, 60, 70, 91, 96, 111–112, 127, 142, 165
homonym 136
Hong Kong Sign Language (HKSL) 42, 50

iconicity 18–21, 55, 67, 126, 130, 134, 149–153, 156, 160–161, 163
incorporation 73
index 14, 16, 43, 45, 47, 70, 79–80, 82, 97, 118, 130, 137, 140, 142
Indopakistani Sign Language (IPSL) 40, 128
inflection 13–14, 20, 56, 74, 80, 124, 127, 133, 135–136, 141–142, 160
Irish Sign Language (ISL) 1–2, 4–8, 10–14, 16–18, 20–24, 27–30, 49, 53, 56–58, 63–66, 69–71, 74–75, 78–85, 89, 92, 94–97, 99, 101–102, 109, 111–115, 129, 132–146, 148–151, 153–165
Israeli Sign Language (IsSL) 30, 43, 45, 48, 61, 127, 149

language mode continuum 112
Langue des Signes Française (LSF) 4
Langue des Signes Québécois (LSQ) 11, 128–129
Lautsprachbegleitende Gebärden (LBG) 6
lexical class 16, 133, 139–142, 144, 151, 154–156, 163–164
Lingua dei Segni Italina (LIS) 39, 43, 50, 128
Llengua des Signes Catalana (LSC) 35, 50

manual 1, 7, 24–26, 28, 36, 45–50, 52–56, 58–60, 64, 70–79, 81–84, 86–92, 95–101, 103, 150–153, 162–163
Mauritian Sign Language (MSL) 53, 56, 64
metalinguistic 81, 83, 120, 157, 162, 164
modifier phrase 137, 146
monolingualism 7, 112, 163
morphological complexity 2, 53, 59, 114–115, 127, 145–148, 155–156, 164
morphosyntax 20, 47, 52, 115, 118–119, 123, 125–126, 128, 132, 134–135, 139–141, 145–147, 155, 157, 164
motivated 18, 130
mouth action 61, 79, 85, 94–95, 98–99, 101, 103, 105–107, 109–110, 114, 145, 163

Nederlandse Gebarentaal (NGT) 2, 38, 40, 53, 57, 59–60, 62, 71, 75, 92, 111, 162–163
(non-)concatenative 8, 21–23, 47, 60, 78, 84, 92, 100, 127, 157
non-manual 5, 22–32, 34, 37–40, 42–44, 46–47, 49–50, 58, 60–61, 67, 80, 113, 132
Norwegian Sign Language (NSL) 60, 78
noun 43, 74, 114, 117–121, 124–125, 129, 147, 160

object 13–16, 20, 22, 33–34, 42, 52, 64, 74, 80–81, 133, 149
oral-aural 11, 163, 165
oralism 9, 11, 51, 55, 57, 59, 68–69, 94–95, 100, 108–109, 112, 165

Part-of-speech (PoS) 114–115, 119, 121, 132–133, 155, 157, 160, 164
personal story 96
pragmatics 26, 32, 40, 43, 45–47, 74, 123, 157, 160–161, 164
predicate 29, 50, 69, 122, 125, 133–134, 136–137, 140, 142, 144, 146, 156, 158–161, 164
progressive spreading 62–63, 78–79, 96, 98
pronoun 12–13, 15, 42, 48, 79, 118–119, 125, 128, 130–131
prosodic binding 61–63, 80
prosody 22, 31–32, 35, 40, 46–48, 61–63, 79–81, 160, 162
prototype theory 120–121, 125, 128

reduced mouthing 60, 83, 100, 103
referential phrase 137, 146
regressive spreading 62, 78–80, 96, 98–99, 101, 104
relative pronoun 42

semantically empty mouth gesture 89
semantic congruence 71, 79, 95, 98, 103, 157, 161–162
semantic redundancy 56, 72, 162
Signed English 11, 135
Signs of Ireland Corpus (SOI) 2, 5, 66–68, 71, 75, 84, 91–96, 103, 114–115, 139, 162
simultaneity 8, 21–23, 47, 60, 78, 84, 92, 100, 157
simultaneous compound 60, 78
sociolinguistic(s) 2, 5, 8, 55, 66, 71, 93–94, 102, 114, 145, 162–163
spreading 35, 39, 47, 49, 51, 54, 58, 60–63, 77–81, 83–84, 92, 96, 98–99, 101, 104, 161
storyline 81–83
subject 5, 13, 20, 29, 31, 33, 80, 120, 122, 149
Swedish Sign Language (SSL) 52–53, 59, 62, 80, 92
syntactic category 137, 139, 141–142, 146, 158
syntax 13, 25, 28, 30, 32, 35–40, 46–48, 58, 60, 62, 69–70, 115–119, 122–125, 127–130, 132–146, 148–149, 155–158, 160–161, 164

tense 44, 54, 75, 86, 89, 123–125, 129

tone 23, 47, 61–62

topic 1, 18–19, 21, 23, 29–30, 40–43, 50–51, 64–65, 123, 126, 129, 131, 160–161, 165

topic marker 30, 50

Turkish Sign Language (TSL) 50

typology 2, 4–5, 64, 66, 71, 83–84, 92, 115, 126, 131, 133, 154–155, 157, 162

valency 120, 134, 159

variation 2, 7–8, 10, 53, 57, 59–60, 62, 68, 95, 120, 129, 162–163

visual-gestural 1, 11, 24, 110, 139, 150, 154

word class 2, 59, 69–70, 80, 93, 115–116, 118–120, 122–128, 130–134, 144, 148–150, 154–157, 162, 164

Kolibri 360 GmbH
Ferdinand-Jühlke-Straße 7
99095 Erfurt, Deutschland
produktsicherheit@kolibri360.de